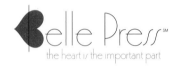

Belle Press℠

the heart is the important part

"I **am** a survivor."

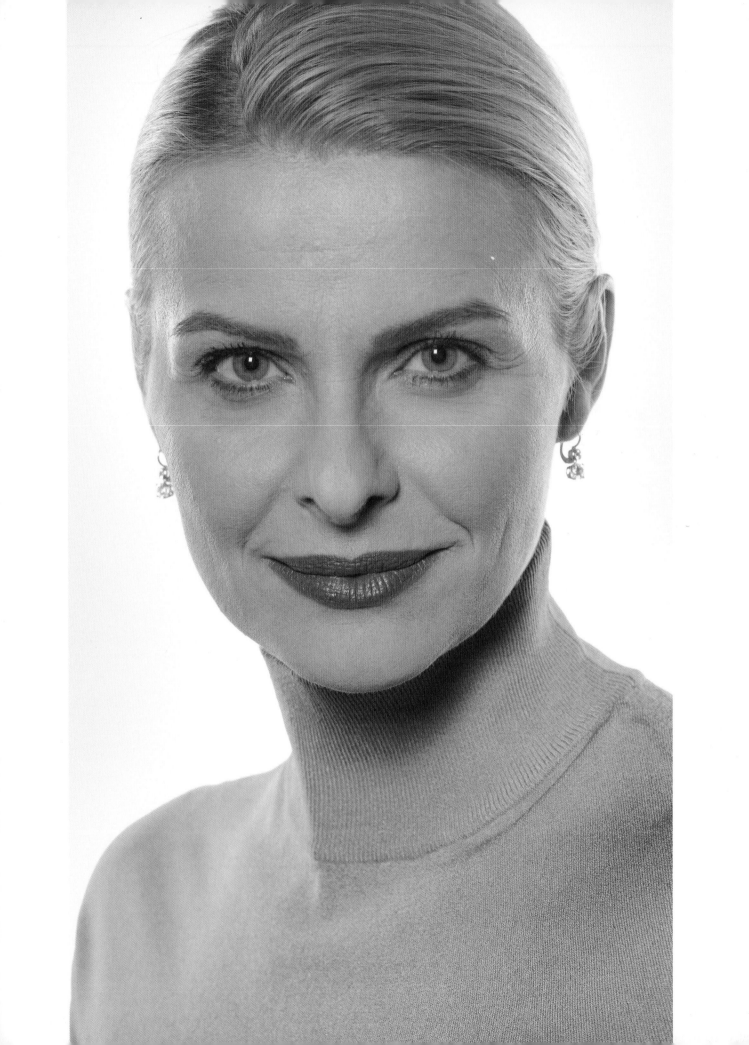

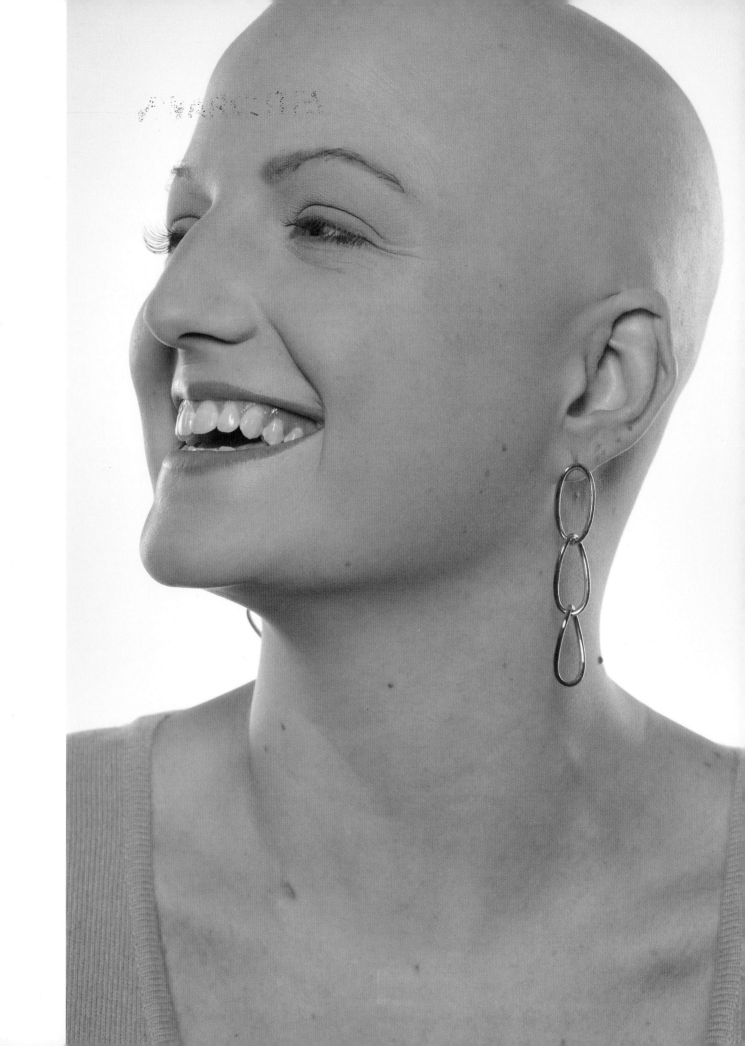

Lori Ovitz

with

Joanne Kabak

Cover Photo: Lori Ovitz
Design and Art Direction: Taylor Bruce Associates
Photography of Cancer Patients and Survivors: Tom Maday
Photo Styling: Bill Zbaren
Product Photography: Kritsada/Krantz Studio
Flowers Donated by: Ronsley Special Events
Jewelry Provided by: Sydney Garber
Printed in the USA by: Lake County Press

Facing The Mirror With Cancer

Visit our website at www.facingthemirror.org

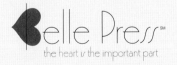

the heart is the important part

A Belle Press Book
Chicago, Illinois

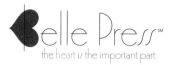
the heart is the important part

Chicago, Illinois

Belle Press is a service mark of Belle Press, LLC.
Facing The Mirror With Cancer and *Facing The
Mirror* are trademarks of Facing The Mirror
With Cancer, LLC.

For information regarding book purchases,
call Facing The Mirror With Cancer, LLC
at 312-214-3545 or visit our website at
www.facingthemirror.org.

Library of Congress Control Number:
2004100851

ISBN: 0-9748938-0-3

First Edition 2004

The content of this book is not intended to
be substituted for medical advice. Whenever
in question, always check with your doctor or
healthcare professional.

"I witnessed *Facing The Mirror With Cancer* begin with a call
to service, and saw it dance into reality with a heartfelt
commitment and a lot of work and faith. Watching this inkling
become a living, full-fledged book has been a joy for me.
Helping to weave the tapestry of *Facing The Mirror With Cancer* by
connecting caring and creative people to one another was a
task laced with synchronicity and grace. There is a sprinkle of
loving magic in Lori Ovitz, in this project, and in healing beauty
and the hope it offers us all."

– Julia A. Bondi, PhD

To Bruce, Kimmy, and Brynn
for showing me every day how to
live, love, and laugh.

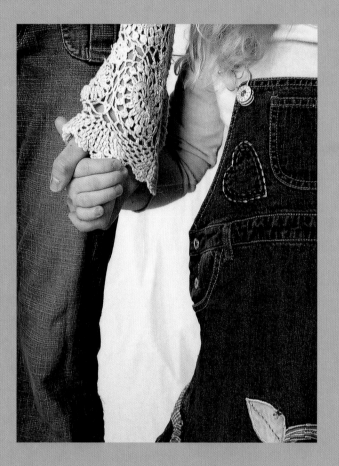

To my mom and dad for instilling in me your values, your
love, and the freedom to choose who I want to be…
You've been behind me every step of the way.

To my mother-in-law for raising her son
to be the extraordinary man he has become.
Isadore, you'd be so proud.

Photograph by Sher Sussman

To all the people who wanted their expressions shared… to help the next… to make it easier… to make a difference.

Acknowledgments

My deepest thanks to everyone involved in this book. Each of you saw the need... and had the commitment... to make a difference for people with cancer.

Bruce – You believed in me and the need for this book so much you became the publisher! You've never forgotten where you've been, where life has taken you, or where you are now. You are a unique man.

Lance Armstrong – For supporting my book, for being a true hero, and for supporting the people who are the real heroes.

Bobbi Brown – Thank you for giving the best advice to a naïve makeup artist in 1984. Thank you for supporting this book 20 years later.

Gina Graci, PhD, and Stephanie Gutz, MSW, LCSW – For acknowledging the importance that makeup can have for cancer patients in improving their lives.

Dr. John T. Grayhack, MD – For being an incredible doctor now and 35 years ago.

Dr. Anthony J. Schaeffer, MD – For being such an instrumental voice and wonderful friend.

Dr. Diane Berson, assistant professor of dermatology at Weill Medical College of Cornell University in New York City – Thank you for answering all of our skin care questions.

Meryl Moss, my publicist – For diving into this project with full force! Thanks for being you – you are my mediamuscle.

Joanne Kabak – Thank you for capturing my voice on paper, for believing in me enough to trust me, for giving your heart and talents to this project.

Susan Maman – A special thank-you for sharing your photographs and your story so openly and beautifully. I received the true beauty – your friendship!

Dr. Abbie Roth, MD – Your support and enthusiasm have been tremendous.

Julia Bondi, PhD – For supporting me through this whole project and for keeping me balanced.

Susan Keeler – For helping create the Belle Press logo on a napkin while we were having dinner at Gene & Georgetti, for sharing the experience of helping to put smiles on the faces of children undergoing cancer treatment, and for being the true definition of friendship.

Doug Bruce and Jared Tekiele of Taylor Bruce Associates, my design team – You captured my true vision of this book and made it a reality, plus!

Tom Maday Photography – You have an amazing ability of capturing the inner and outer beauty of the people you photograph.

Maureen Donlan and Brian Blanchard – Thank you for selflessly sharing your expertise to make a difference for others.

Loretta Wilger-Asmus – For being the dynamo that you are.

Kritsada/Krantz Studio – For transforming a simple product into a work of art.

Linda Nowlin-Dineff Trademark Law, Ltd – For protecting my good name.

Steve Florsheim, Sperling and Slater – For handling all my legal needs.

Hillary Jambor, Michele Fisher, Allison Fiedel, Sarah and Henry King, and Olga Markoff – For all your enormous support. You've each added something special to this book.

Chanda Mehta, LCSW – For giving me the chance to show what I could do for oncology children and adults at University of Chicago Hospital.

Ross Cosmetics – Arden and Earl Edelcup, for all of your support over the years.

Julie Penfield – For all the special things you do running our *Facing The Mirror With Cancer* office.

Mary Catherine "MC" Mortell – Thanks for being you.

Vita and Irma – Thank you for all you do for me and my family.

Rebecca, Sylvia, Angel, Margaret, Loretta, and Renee – For sharing your faces and thoughts to demonstrate how makeup can and does make a difference.

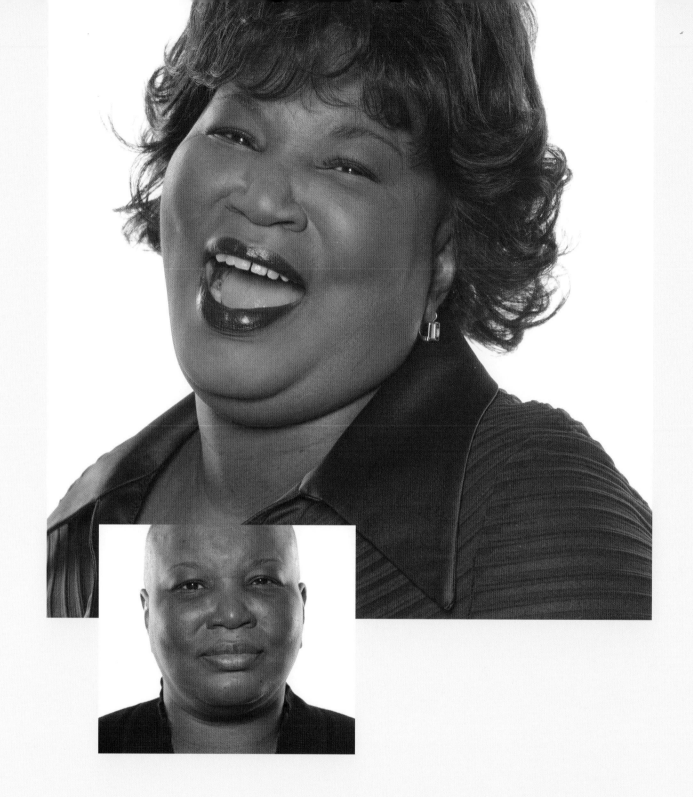

"When people at a charity event I attended kept telling me how beautiful I looked, I told them I had a secret weapon!"

– Lilian C.

Foreword

Just a generation ago, the prognosis for many cancers was often so bleak that cancer patients routinely hid their diagnoses from neighbors, co-workers, friends, and even their families. Turning their backs on a potentially supportive network to spare loved ones from their grim ordeal was often the only control many cancer patients could exert over their fate. Today, research has tremendously advanced not only our understanding of cancer, but also the efficacy of medical treatments. Breakthroughs in science and medical research and the success of cancer-related treatments, including chemotherapy, radiation, and surgery, continue to change the meaning of a cancer diagnosis, yet the physical toll exacted by a battle with cancer remains daunting.

Having known Lori for the past seven years, I have seen the passion that she applies to her craft and the compassion she has for those undergoing cancer therapy. Helping to restore some control to those experiencing the debilitating effects of treatment has inspired Lori to share her passion with her book *Facing The Mirror With Cancer*.

Lori's husband Bruce – a 35-year cancer survivor – is a committed and grateful champion of the people who gave him back his life. Bruce has been a major contributor and enthusiastic fund raiser on behalf of Northwestern University's Department of Urology since 1975.

I commend Lori for sharing her methods to battle the physical effects of treatment and praise Lori and Bruce for making the financial commitment to publish this book. It is no surprise that 50 percent of their personal profits will be donated to cancer research to further the advancement of research technologies so that more people can survive this disease.

– Dr. Anthony J. Schaeffer, MD
Chairman of the Department of Urology
The Feinberg School of Medicine,
Northwestern University.

"You'll be amazed by what you can do when you think you look good. It can actually become contagious."

We don't go through life expecting to get a diagnosis of cancer, and when we do, it can be devastating. It affects us emotionally, socially, physically, and functionally. We can become tearful and sad, lose interest in things we love, and begin to withdraw from life, people, and events. Sometimes the common side effects of treatment such as hair loss or nausea promote anxiety or depression. We begin to cancel appointments, even work engagements, because we just don't look or feel well. It is easy to begin to live day to day because our life has been turned upside down. We don't prepare for cancer because we don't expect it to happen to us.

The security that we once felt within our bodies and the way in which we view the world is threatened. The disease and its treatment can change how we look and feel about ourselves and have devastating effects on our emotional well-being. How we look at ourselves in the mirror is now different. For example, hair loss, skin coloring changes, and the inability to have healthy-looking nails become a temporary part of who we are and how others begin to see us. I have heard patients say, "I didn't realize the cure could be worse than the cancer." Cancer *does not* have to rob you of your self-esteem, confidence, or beauty. The diagnosis of cancer affects people of all ages and races, and it affects both men and women. It is scary to know that you have cancer and have to begin treatment. Everyone has heard about the side effects of treatment – the good news is that many of the side effects can be managed.

Physical appearance is important to one's mental health. People judge us by how we look, and often how we look affects the way we feel. Have you ever gone out and bought a new outfit that you knew looked fantastic on you? You know the boost of confidence and the rise in self-esteem associated with looking good. If you look good, you feel good. This principle holds true for anyone facing a life-threatening illness. Taking care of your looks is taking care of yourself and is leading you toward a healthy lifestyle. If you look good, you will feel better emotionally, and this emotional boost can do wonders for your body. You'll be able to manage pain more effectively, and depression and anxiety levels can decrease. You will want to reclaim your life in every way possible.

Many of my patients voice concerns about returning to work or are concerned about how their physical appearance may affect their children. They often say, "I just don't want people to know that I am sick. I don't want to be treated differently." We take pride in our appearance, and the side effects of cancer treatment affect people differently. Many people complain that they do not look like themselves, that they have become a different person. Many parents become concerned that if they look like they have cancer, then their children will become frightened. These concerns are normal and appropriate. The good news is that no one has to feel this way. You can begin facing the mirror confidently with cancer and embrace life again. This guidebook will help you face the physical side effects of cancer and treatment. It will show you how to enhance your beauty, joy, happiness, love, and live life to the fullest.

We all begin journeys in life, and we all choose different paths. Some journeys are filled with obstacles we didn't necessarily plan for or expect. George Strait, a famous country music singer, wrote a song titled, *Living and Living Well*. The song brilliantly illustrates that there is a difference between staying alive and living well. This principle applies to everyone, especially individuals afflicted with a life-threatening illness. Lori Ovitz has created a way for you to embark on your journey and face the mirror. She offers every person facing cancer ways to restore and enhance their quality of life. I encourage everyone with cancer to embrace life and face the mirror. I think you'll be overjoyed with the outcome.

– Gina Graci, PhD
Director, Psychosocial Oncology
Assistant Professor of Psychiatry
Accredited Behavioral Sleep Medicine Specialist (AASM)
Robert H. Lurie Comprehensive Cancer Center
Northwestern University Feinberg School of Medicine

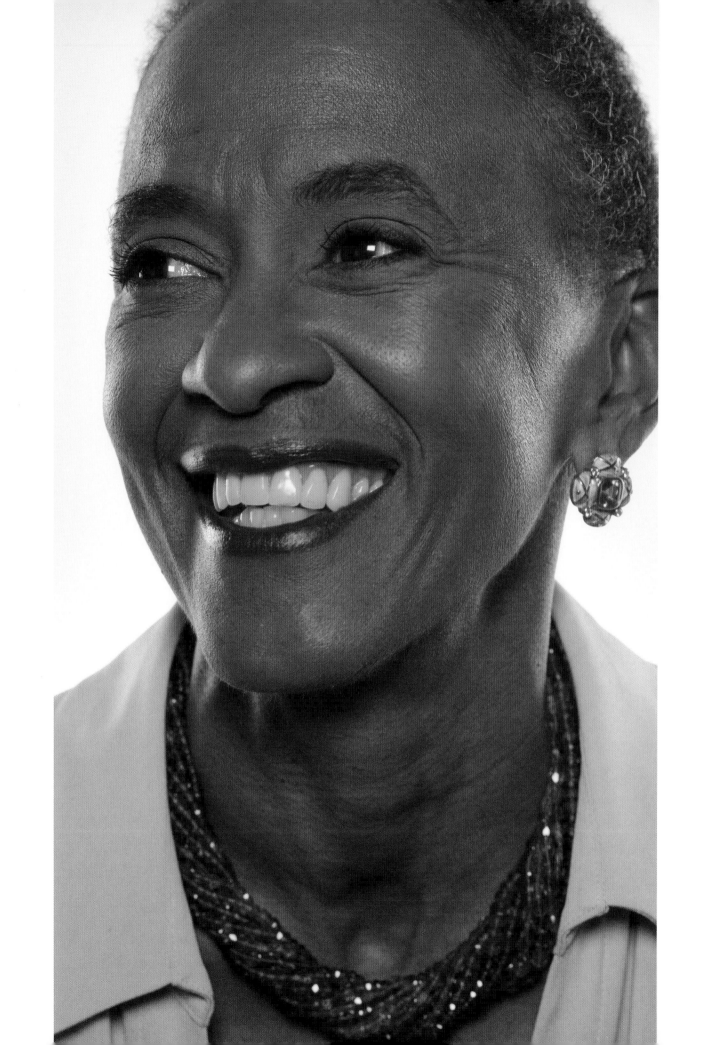

Introduction
Lori Ovitz

After I taught Debbie how to use makeup to change the visible side effects of cancer treatments, she looked like herself again on the outside. But there was something more. She also felt like herself again on the inside, with more confidence and energy. Watching her transformation helped me to forever change my thinking about makeup.

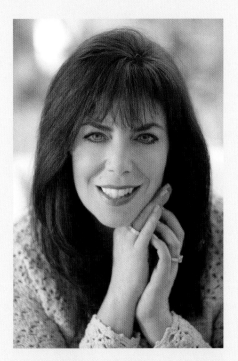

Photograph of Lori Ovitz by Kritsada/Krantz Studio

Before I met Debbie or any of the many cancer patients I've worked with, being a professional makeup artist to the stars was my passionate goal. And I didn't let anything discourage me – even the comments of the owner of the makeup salon where I first worked as a junior assistant. In 1983 when I shared my dreams with her, she snapped back at me, *"I'll grow tomatoes when you make it doing makeup for print, advertising, and television."*

Instead of giving up, I went on to learn the tricks of the trade so well that in 1986 I signed with a top Chicago agency, David and Lee (now owned by the Ford Modeling Agency.) And I received great career advice from one of today's most respected makeup professionals, Bobbi Brown. She gave me time on the phone when I was an unknown but highly driven young woman, committed to succeeding and motivated to learn everything. What she told me in that five-minute conversation set me on my path as a professional makeup artist. When I turned to her with my intention to write this book, she once again gave me her support. Her endorsement was invaluable to me at a time when this book was in its planning stage.

During my 20 years as a professional makeup artist working with beautiful models and well-known celebrities, nothing has given me greater satisfaction than working with cancer patients. My interests began to shift when I volunteered at a cancer center. I saw that along with medical issues, for every patient there is a complex emotional side to cancer. I understood how research has made enormous progress and that even as they fight the disease, people with cancer now continue to go out into the world to work, raise a family, and have a social life. But one of the things that can hold them back is the discomfort they feel about the changes in their appearance. These aesthetic changes may be temporary, but they can feel devastating.

I knew it didn't have to be this way. Makeup is an accessible, inexpensive way to make significant changes in your appearance. It can lessen the effects of treatments on your skin, features, and hair and restore you as closely as possible to the way you looked before cancer. I began to develop techniques that really work for side effects such as loss of eyebrow and eyelash hair and for camouflaging skin damage.

The most rewarding part of doing this work has been seeing how people's attitude and courage grow more positive as they learn to take control of their appearance. Many studies show a link between positive attitude and improved outcomes for people dealing with cancer. Makeup will not cure a cancer, but makeup makes it a whole lot easier to face the mirror.

The tremendous gratitude I've received from each patient I've worked with at the Robert H. Lurie Comprehensive Cancer Center at Northwestern University has inspired me to write this book. I often think of the many people I've taught, like the corporate executive who was so concerned that when she went back to work, everyone in her office would see right away that she had cancer. The last thing she needed was to feel exposed or pitied. What she needed most was to walk into work with the sense of dignity, control, and energy that comes from looking your best no matter how daunting your challenges are. Makeup was able to do that for her, as it has for so many.

A single makeup artist can serve only a limited number of people. A book of techniques that is clear, comprehensive, and written with love can reach huge numbers of cancer patients who need to know this information. The message of the book is, "You can look like yourself." The question it answers is, "How do I do it and where do I begin?"

When many publishers did not want to take a chance with this subject, my husband Bruce, a 35-year cancer survivor himself, and I decided to publish this book ourselves. As someone who has undergone cancer and its treatments, he really understands the reason for the book and is passionate about bringing it to everyone who needs it. Together we created Belle Press. And together we bring to you the message that comes straight from cancer patients who've already benefited from using these techniques: They work.

Best wishes to you during treatment and always,

Lori

"As a health journalist, I was drawn to work with Lori on this book because of her powerful commitment to using her special makeup skills to make a difference for people with cancer. In her photographs, she breaks taboos about showing real people with altered features and without hair. In her words, she knocks down every belief that it's somehow acceptable to feel ashamed by the visible effects of disease and treatment. In every respect, this is a book whose time has come."

— Joanne Kabak, journalist and collaborator with Lori in writing this book

Letter From Susan

Dear Lori,

Rather than write something to you with today's date in mind, I thought you would enjoy reading some excerpts from the sporadic diary I kept during my challenging chemotherapy days.

Among the many trials and tribulations of breast cancer and its treatments is the shock of losing one's hair. For me this was particularly painful, as I have been what you could call a "hair neurotic" for the past 30 years or more. Hair frames the face and is a great part of a woman's beauty. It's one of the first features I notice. I love beautiful hair and can appreciate a great-looking hairstyle.

As my hair began to fall out, I knew I would have to shave it off sooner or later. And one Sunday afternoon, my close friends and I went to do the inevitable. But I didn't have the courage and wasn't mentally ready. Instead I had my hair cut very short, and the hair that was left was hanging on by a thread. In fact I thought if I went downtown and the wind was too strong, the hair on my head would just disappear with the wind.

With the onset of my second chemotherapy treatment, I had only one choice left – to shave my head. Soon the final hour arrived. Brian gently kissed my head and took the razor down the middle first. I shed a few tears, and before I knew it I was completely bald. I looked in the mirror, and initially I was shocked.

I thought I looked so old. But as time wore on, I kept thinking *it's me*. I'm still the same spirit, the same human being, the same wife, the same mother, the same sister, the same friend. I believe that Jordan and Monique were shocked to see their mom bald. The fact that I had breast cancer and was sick and undergoing chemotherapy really set in with the loss of my hair.

I did have a beautiful wig to put on, but I needed something, a new lift, some way to make me feel beautiful even if I didn't have hair. I needed something to give me the confidence to go out in public with a simple hat or scarf. I needed a way to still feel attractive, pretty, soft, and feminine.

That boost of confidence came in the form of acceptance of my situation and not feeling sorry for myself. The boost also came from learning how to apply my makeup and how to deal with the other effects of chemotherapy: the loss of eyelashes and eyebrows, the loss of weight that made my face thinner and my wrinkles more pronounced, and the loss of my normal skin color.

Lori Ovitz's visit enabled me to learn how to apply my makeup in a very short period of time and feel good about my appearance. To this day, I still say to myself as I apply my under-eye concealer, "pat and press gently." Her simple and easy-to-follow guidelines have become a way of life, a routine that has put sunshine back in some very cloudy days and nights. I have tried not to be vain, but the fact remains that I do care about my appearance. I want to look good again. Looking and feeling good are a part of dealing with the many challenges that life during chemotherapy presents. Sometimes just looking good helps you to feel good. I received so many compliments on my face that I truly feel confident about my looks.

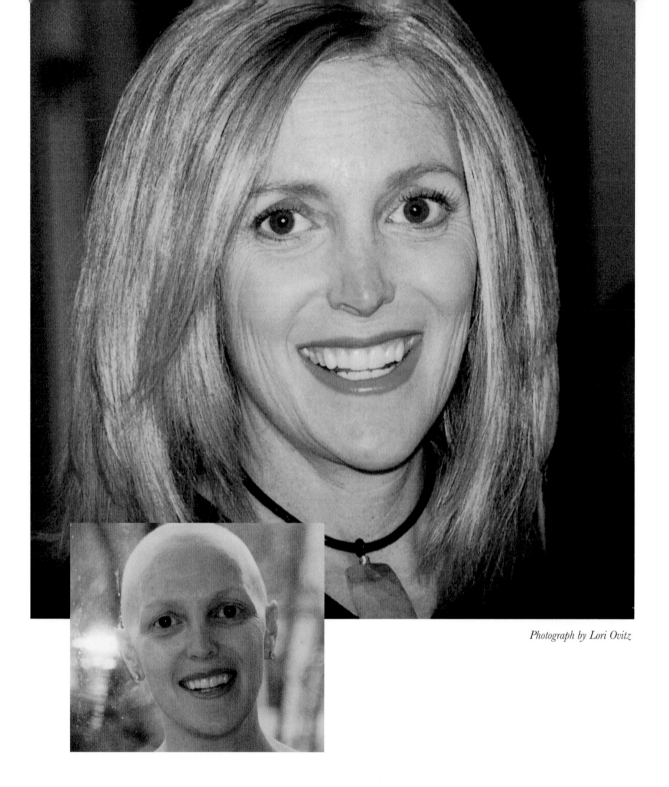

Photograph by Lori Ovitz

"My hair is back, I'm done with treatment, and I still use these techniques! Your tricks helped me look good then, so you can imagine how great I look now!"

– Susan M.

If someone had told me a year ago that I could go to a party with no hair on my head, I would have told them they were out of their mind. It could and would never happen. But I have found the inner strength and courage to do so from a positive attitude, a strong spirit, and confidence in my ability to still feel pretty in spite of it all.

These accomplishments are partially, if not largely, due to my newly acquired makeup skills. I truly believe that every woman undergoing chemotherapy has the opportunity to help herself feel pretty even though her hair is gone. And it takes some expert advice, given with warmth and love, to give one back that lift of confidence.

Lori, I thank you from the bottom of my heart, for giving me all these wonderful tips and insights and helping put that smile back on my face.

Love always, your ever-appreciative friend,
Susan

TABLE OF CONTENTS

Part I – Looking at Makeup in a Different Way

Part II – Makeup: This Is How You Do It

Part III – From Head to Toe

Part IV – Not for Women Only: Techniques for the Special Needs of Men, Children, and Teens

Understanding
Skin Care

Skin Care Basics

Questions and Answers From a
Board-Certified Dermatologist

*"I'm so glad I came to keep Betty company
(during her makeup session.) I've learned so much!"*

– Terry J.

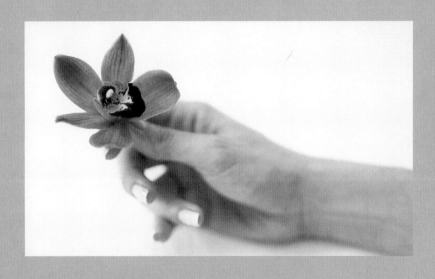

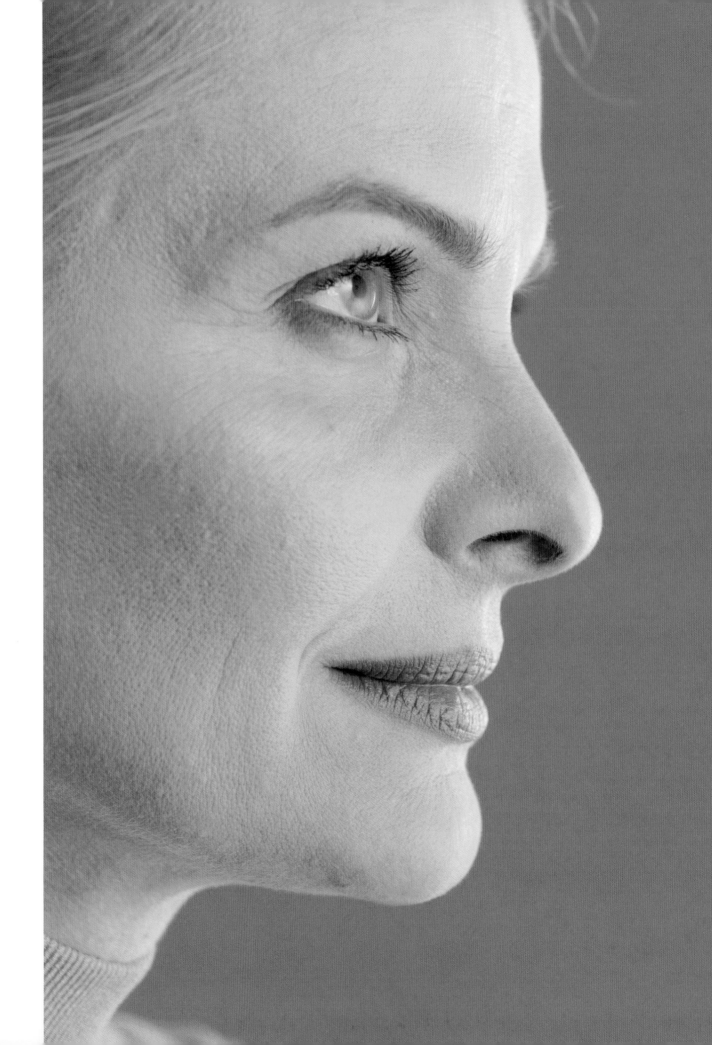

UNDERSTANDING SKIN CARE

Dr. Diane S. Berson, assistant professor of dermatology at Weill Medical College of Cornell University in New York City, answers many of the questions that you may have about how to care for your skin while undergoing chemotherapy and radiation. If you have any concerns or specific questions about your situation, be sure to check with your doctor.

There are many gentle, soothing steps you can take to help your skin feel natural and soft. Since you may be experiencing increased skin sensitivity, you also will want to know how to avoid skin irritation.

Q: What are the best types of skin cleansers to use at this time?

Treat your skin as though it were very sensitive.

- Use mild cleansers such as liquids and bars labeled for sensitive skin.
- Don't scrub.
- Don't use harsh products or rough washcloths.
- Keep water at a moderate temperature.
- To dry your skin, pat it gently – don't rub it.

Your skin will feel so good and refreshed!

Q: Do you recommend using a toner?

If you have oily skin, use a toner. Choose a product that contains salicylic acid.

Q: What kind of moisturizer is best?

Select a moisturizer with emollients such as glycerin or petrolatum. Stay away from products containing fragrances and additives since they can irritate sensitive skin.

Q: What suggestions do you have for acne?

For mild acne, use a mild, antibacterial cleanser. Gently pat your face dry. Apply toner in the T-zone, going from the forehead down the middle of the face. Add a light moisturizer.

If acne persists or is severe, check with your doctor.

Q: Is it OK to have a facial?

Yes – but because your skin is sensitive, there may be changes to your usual routine:

- Choose a facial that gives you a soothing, gentle cleansing.

- Avoid extreme temperatures.

- Do not use steam treatments.

- Avoid any probing of the skin.

Q: Is it OK to have electrolysis or waxing?

It's best to check with your doctor. If you do use either procedure, test an area of your skin first to make sure you can tolerate it. And have any treatments done with extra gentleness.

Q: What is preferred: bathing or showering?

Both are fine. Here are my favorite tips:

- Keep the water temperature moderate.

- Use a mild cleanser for the body.

- If bathing, soak in the tub for about 10 minutes, then add a bath oil. Your skin will absorb the oil much better after soaking!

- Oatmeal products for the bath are wonderfully soothing.

- After leaving a bath or shower, pat your skin gently to dry. Don't rub it!

- Immediately apply an emollient-rich moisturizer all over your skin – dampness helps skin absorb moisturizer.

Q: What can you do if skin feels itchy, inflamed, or irritated?

Here is "Dr. Berson's favorite recipe":

Mix together:
½ bowl of milk
½ bowl of water
ice cubes

Dip a washcloth in the mixture, wring it out, and put it on the affected area. Then apply moisturizer mixed with a little anti-inflammatory cortisone cream (available over the counter). Enjoy the soothing feeling!

Q: Which is preferred: shaving with an electric razor or with a blade?

An electric razor is a much better choice because there is a risk of nicks, cuts, and bleeding when using a razor blade. If you must use a blade, be extremely careful. And always protect your skin with a shaving cream or gel for sensitive skin.

Q: What about sunscreen?

It's a must! Since the skin is in a more sensitive state, whenever any part of your skin is exposed to the sun it has to be protected.

Best choices: Apply SPF 30 to the skin. Use a product that provides both UVB and UVA protection.

Q: Can you use makeup to cover scars?

Yes – as long as the scars are healed, and there's no longer an open wound. To apply makeup, gently pat the area. Be extra gentle when removing makeup.

Q: When can you expect dryness and redness to go away?

Typically, the skin improves in about four to six weeks after treatment ends. In the meantime, you can always use makeup to cover!

Since everyone's skin is different, it's important to check with your doctor about any specific questions. But I hope my recommendations have helped you. It can feel so good to have skin that's been soothed and cared for gently!

Getting Started

Practical Considerations

Organizing and Evaluating
What You Have at Home

*"Taking the time to do my makeup in the morning gave me
strength and security throughout the day."*

– Jane C.

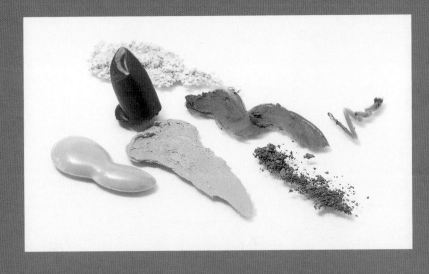

"Where do I begin? I've got a lot of makeup at home, but I'm not sure if it's the right stuff or what to do with it. And it's hard to figure all this out at a time when I just don't feel like myself."

– Celia F.

This book is for you – designed to support and guide you so you can comfortably apply makeup to address the changes you've been going through. You will learn exactly how to use makeup as a corrective tool – calmly, with confidence, and in private. I know it's a big step. When people call me for a makeup session, I hear the quiver in their voices. And then I hear that quiver disappear as they begin to see how well makeup works and that it is possible to do it themselves.

I'm so glad you've decided to take this book in hand and gain as much control as you can over your appearance. The key is knowing how to use cosmetics as a corrective tool. The benefits of makeup come from two sources: having the right tools and using the right techniques. I will guide you in gathering the products you already own and in evaluating how you can use them in different ways. I will walk you through the items you need and the techniques that are most effective so you can do a fabulous job of applying makeup on your own.

Each chapter of the book is designed to support the chapters that follow. The reason I've put the lessons in a certain order is to build the groundwork for your whole look to come together. The lessons are also designed to stand alone, so that depending on your needs and your time, you can do the steps individually.

This is your time to give a gift to yourself – learning how to use makeup so that you look like yourself – naturally. Makeup is magic, and it's fun. No matter how tired or stressed you may be, I encourage you to enjoy the experience. Allow yourself to feel pleasure in the brightness of the colors, the softness of the brushes, the gentleness of the powders and creams.

Choose a space where you can sit down comfortably and spread out your supplies. Add good lighting and a mirror. And set aside enough time, uninterrupted, to learn these techniques step-by-step.

At the beginning, it seems like a lot to learn. Be patient. Once you've mastered these lessons, you'll have plenty of opportunity to do your makeup on the fly. You can do it anywhere! I've applied makeup on clients in treatment rooms in the hospital and at kitchen tables in their homes. The luxury of doing makeup is not just the pleasing end result, but the whole process of creating your look, step-by-step, with your own hands.

Important note: Please remember to always check with your doctor if you have any questions or concerns about any tool, technique, or ingredient before you use it.

It's important for you to get medical advice to find out whether it's safe to apply a makeup product and, if so, when you can start using it. This is especially true after surgery, or if you have any type of fresh wound, scar, or other alteration to your skin. Also, be sure to ask about ingredients you should avoid.

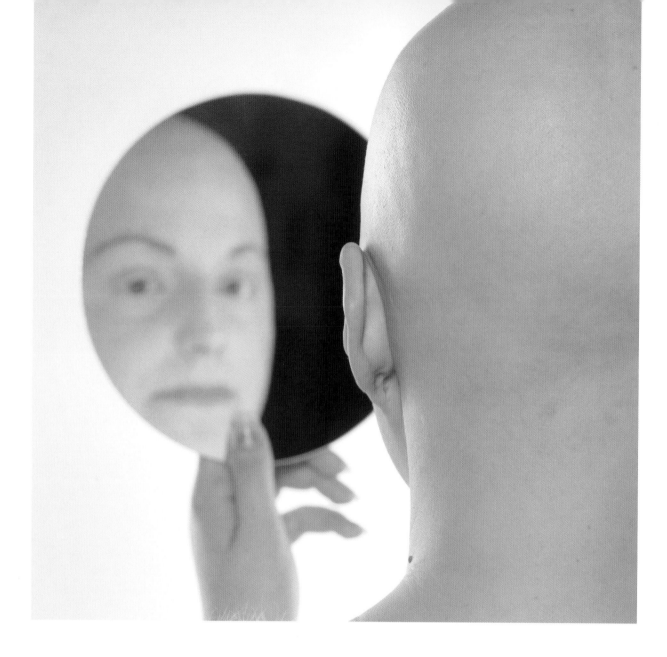

Practical Considerations

- Hygiene. Good hygiene is a must! At a time when you are particularly susceptible to infections, simple steps like washing your hands and using cleaned and disinfected tools are an essential part of your makeup routine.

- Light. Natural daylight is great for working on your makeup. When using artificial light, make sure it's as close to natural daylight as possible.

- Mirror. Everyone seems to have a favorite mirror for doing close-up work, whether it's the one on the medicine chest, at a makeup table or bureau, or one that you hold in your hand. Choose the mirror that works best for you. Please note: Magnifying mirrors are great for certain purposes, but they can distort images.

Organizing and Evaluating

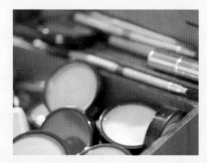

A great way to begin your work is to take out all your makeup products, even the ones you never use, and spread them out. Discard anything that appears to be old – that is, if you can't remember where and when you got it, don't like the way it looks or smells, or see that it is cracked or dusty. If a product is of uncertain quality, do not use it. If you have a brush you like but that appears questionable, you can carefully clean and disinfect it instead of throwing it out.

Next, sort your makeup in piles – one pile for blushes, one for foundations, one for eye shadows, etc.

Evaluate what you have. Some of the items may no longer be your favorites, but you can use them to mix colors and end up with a new shade. Throughout the book, we'll be looking at many such products in a new light.

"Makeup g

the stre

past the mirror

ave me
ngth to go
without fear."

— *Cynthia S.*

Effective Tools

All About the Tools You Use

"My friends joked that I finally learned how to put on my makeup well."

— Danielle W.

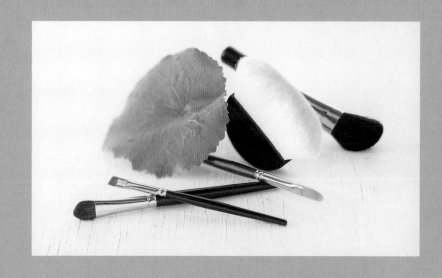

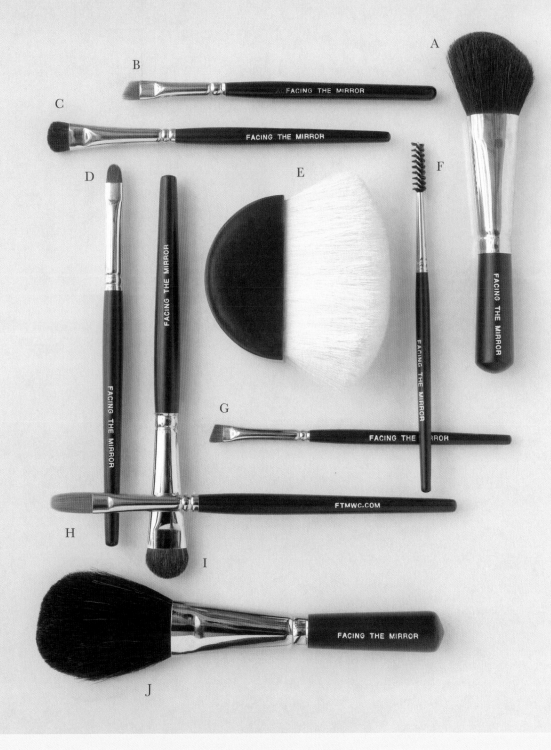

Types of Brushes:

A. *Blush* B. *Eye Liner* C. *Eye Shadow (detail)* D. *Lip* E. *Gentlemen's Powder* F. *Eyebrow Comb*
G. *Brow* H. *Camouflage* I. *Eye Shadow* J. *Powder*

One of the most extraordinary aspects of writing this book has been the amazing people I've met. Some have come into my life for the first time, but others, like Loretta Wilger-Asmus, are people I've known for years. When I first met Loretta, she was one of the world's top models, and I worked with her as a professional makeup artist. Twenty years later, she is a model for this book, showing how you can look your best while battling cancer and beyond.

– Lori

I am a cancer survivor. I used to model for Versace, appear with Cindy Crawford and Imam, and be photographed for catalogues like Neiman Marcus. Then I opened my own business called Looks, to train young men and women in the art of becoming a top model. My life had been glamorous, but in March 2000, I felt my body telling me something was wrong. I went to my doctor and got back a diagnosis I wasn't expecting: adno-cervical and squamous cell carcinomas.

It was so frightening. I didn't know what was going to happen, and I was so upset I couldn't think straight. Fortunately, I had listened to my body early on. I was directed to a wonderful oncologist, Dr. Ronald Potkuhl at Loyola University. Two surgeries and waiting for results took a big toll on me. I lost 25 pounds and most of my hair. It took an entire year to get my health and energy back.

Fully recovered, I've returned to my life with a deeper understanding of how devastating a cancer diagnosis is and how important it is to retain a sense of dignity and a measure of control over our looks during and after treatment. That's why I'm honored to be a part of this book and to use my image, my words, and my personal experience to encourage you to express your own natural beauty no matter what the challenge. I am confident the tools and techniques of *Facing The Mirror With Cancer* can help you do it.

– Loretta Wilger-Asmus

Effective Tools

Part II: Makeup: This Is How You Do It
Camouflage

"I don't want to wear my diagnosis on my sleeve."

– Martina F.

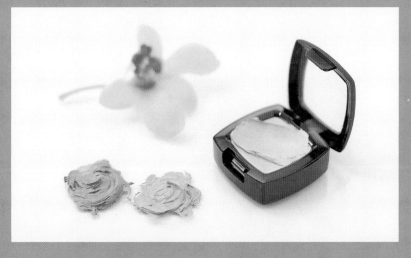

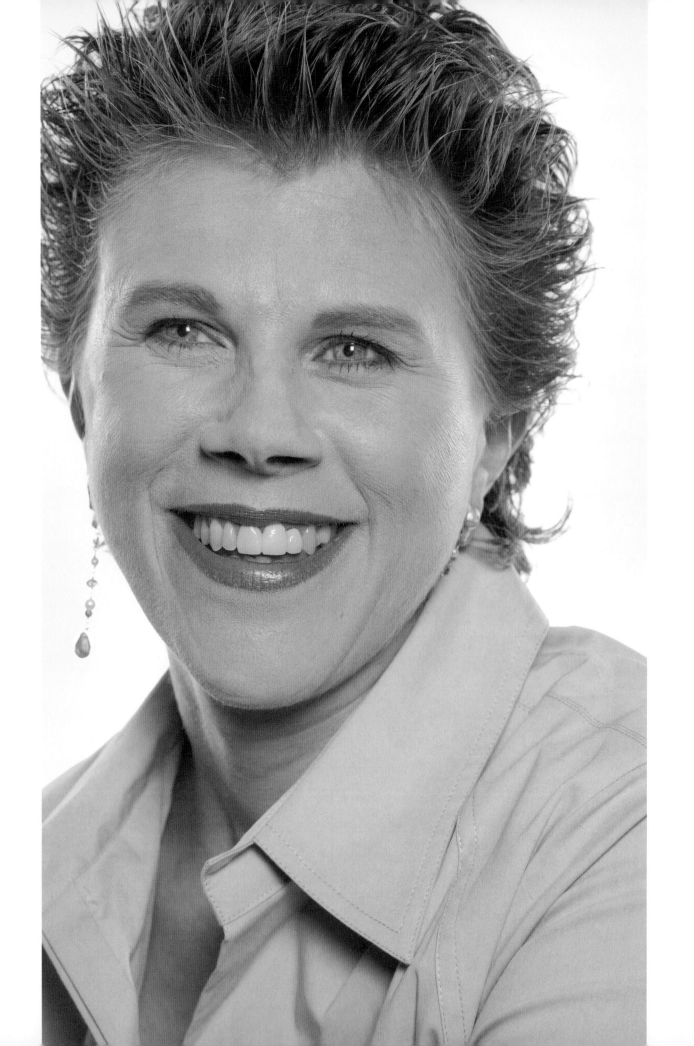

CAMOUFLAGE

For some people, the thick consistency of camouflage makeup is a turn-off. Others feel nervous about applying camouflage themselves because they fear their efforts won't look professional enough, and they'll end up drawing even more attention to an area they want to hide. But the truth about camouflage is this: It works. In this chapter you will learn how to choose the right tone to match your skin and how to apply it so that it covers any imperfection you are concerned about. Rest assured, no one will have to know your secret!

Of all the makeup products available, think of camouflage as the magical tool that is different from the products you use to cover up minor imperfections. Camouflage is used to hide deeper imperfections such as scars, darker discolorations, and other alterations to areas of your skin. Its density makes it ideal for this task. Especially during treatments for cancer, you may have imperfections in your skin that you never had before. Now they are appearing as part of the treatment and healing process, and you can use the tools and techniques of makeup to hide them effectively. Unlike other types of makeup, camouflage is designed to cover up a specific spot and not to be spread over a wide area. It can be used on other parts of the body as well as on the face.

Just a reminder: Camouflage is not a medical treatment, it's strictly a cosmetic coverup. You are not going to be getting rid of a mark, you are going to hide it. When you wash the camouflage off, the mark will still be there. But by using camouflage as a tool during this time, you can change your looks back to more closely resemble the natural you.

What Makes Camouflage Makeup Different

Camouflage has a thicker consistency than foundation. It acts like a double protection for your skin. And it shouldn't be used for any other purpose than hiding imperfections. For example, you wouldn't use camouflage as a highlighter around the eyes to brighten them, but you would use it around the eyes if you had scarring and discoloration in that area.

Another major difference is that camouflage comes in fewer colors than foundation. Also, unlike foundation, camouflage makeup should be water-resistant. This is vital to make sure any marks are covered all day, no matter what activity you engage in, including swimming.

How to Pick Out the Best Camouflage for You

Most camouflage makeup comes in a variety of tones, and the one you choose should be the same tone as your foundation. (If you are planning on not wearing foundation, make sure the camouflage matches your skin tone.) Don't select a camouflage makeup that greatly changes your skin color, thinking that's what makes camouflage work. No! Since this is the first step in concealing imperfections, you want to make sure that the match to your skin tone is as close as possible.

To test whether a color is right for you, use your finger or a sponge to dab a bit of product in the area you want to conceal. Press-pat it on until it becomes invisible. (You'll often hear me refer to the press-pat technique; a detailed description with photos of how to do it is included in the following section on camouflage technique.)

If the color sticks out after several press-pat motions, then the shade is either too dark or too light. Move on to test another shade. When you find one that disappears into your skin, you'll know you have selected the right color to cover your imperfections. A well-chosen color will result in a very pleasing illusion – the spot has vanished!

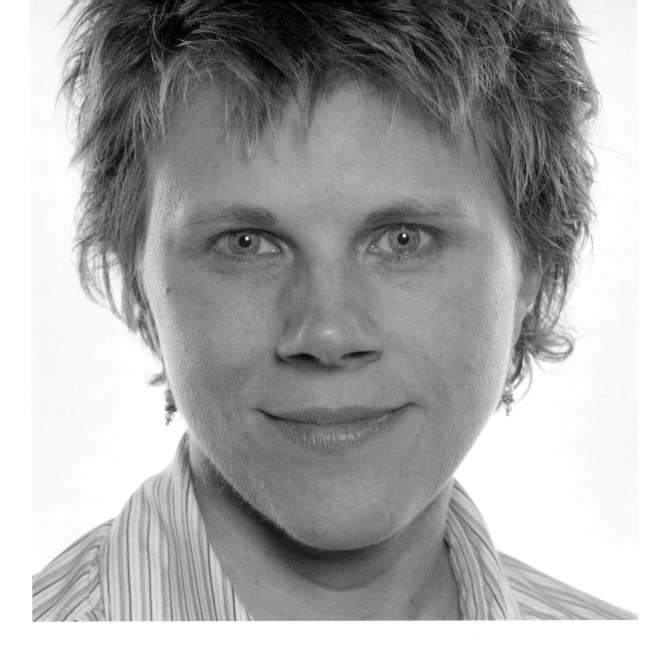

Camouflage Technique

- Use your finger, a sponge, or a concealer brush, depending on the size of the area where you are applying camouflage.

- Apply camouflage with a little dab. Gently press-pat the camouflage into the area you want to conceal.

- Use the press-pat technique until the camouflage is totally blended in with your skin. This technique is important in getting the thick camouflage to effectively cover an area without clumping or appearing too light or too dark. If you press-pat, you will zero in on the area you want to conceal. If you rub it in, the camouflage will spread out over a much wider area. Try both techniques on your hand, and you'll see the difference.

Camouflage

In detail, here is the press-pat technique:

1. Gently pat the makeup onto the area you want to cover.

2. Press it on.

3. Then, continue to press-pat, press-pat. The motion is kind of a "hop-a-long."

4. Always remember to be gentle.

5. Tap softly to blend it in. Do not rub or smear it into your skin.

6. Repeat until well-blended.

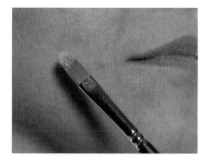

• If you wear foundation, your next step is to apply foundation on top of the camouflage using the press-pat motion. Now you will have two layers of protection, both of them blended in with the rest of your skin. Note: Camouflage can also be worn without foundation.

• If there are small marks on parts of your body other than your face, apply camouflage in the same way as described above. Then apply a setting powder to help the camouflage stay in place. If you are working on a larger area, apply the setting powder with a large fluff brush.

The reason I encourage you to try camouflage is that I have worked with so many clients who start out wary but end up realizing how easy camouflage can be to apply when they follow these techniques. Most of all, they feel better about being in public because imperfections are simply not visible.

*"I never thought I could look
this good again."*

– Rebecca T.

Foundation

"Thanks to teaching my wife about makeup, you gave her back her self-esteem. She hasn't felt this positive about herself for quite a while."

– Joseph T.

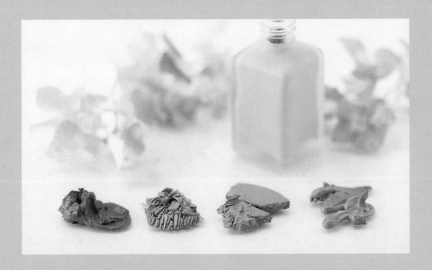

"While undergoing cancer treatment, you may feel like you're losing your sense of identity, which comes from losing the appearance you've always known. Being able to help someone regain his or her normal appearance is an especially important part of recovery. If only my mom could have had that opportunity at the time she was diagnosed with cancer. I was only four years old, and I still remember seeing her when she returned home from the hospital. How thin and pale she looked, all of her hair gone – not like herself at all. At the time, however, there was no one to teach her techniques of makeup application and hair styling to mask the effects of cancer therapy. My mom is a strong woman, and she remains a role model to me in going forward with life no matter the obstacles. Your attitude can make a world of difference, letting you walk back into the world with dignity."

– Dr. Abbie Roth, Obstetrician/Gynecologist in private practice at Northwestern Memorial Hospital in Chicago, clinical instructor at Northwestern University Medical School

INTRODUCTION TO FOUNDATION

Start by evaluating what foundation products you already have at home. It's likely your collection includes free samples that were previously not appropriate for your particular skin type. In thinking about what works for your skin now, describe your skin and determine what, if anything, has changed.

- Is your skin tone different?

- Is your skin texture more dry or more oily?

- Is your skin more sensitive?

With so many different kinds of foundation on the market today, it can be difficult to choose the right one. Ask yourself: Is my skin balanced, dry, or oily? That is what all the different options come down to. Sure, you can get products that are very specific and zero in on combinations of skin types. But unless you identify the basic condition of your skin as it is right now, you could end up with the wrong product and disappointing results.

Shop around for foundation until you find the right formula for you. It will look and act like a second skin. When you're using the right product, no one will be able to tell you're wearing it. That's the point!

Choosing a Foundation

- Color: Match the color to your skin tone to achieve the ideal match. A big mistake is to overcompensate. If you think you're too pale, don't get foundation that's darker. You'll end up looking *too* dark! It doesn't work!

- Texture: Match the product to the present condition of your skin. For example, if your skin has become much drier than it normally is, switch to a more moisturizing foundation. And if your skin has become oily, then it's time for a water-based foundation.

Selecting Color

- Apply a test sample of foundation to your forehead to see if the color blends. If it seems to disappear, and you can't see where the foundation begins or ends, then you have selected the right color.

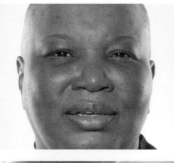

- Always test the color of foundation on your forehead. If you test color on your jawline, the top of your hand, or the back of your wrist, I guarantee you are not comparing it to the same shade as your face. Those areas get different amounts of sun exposure, and if you base your choice on any area other than your face, the color won't blend in naturally.

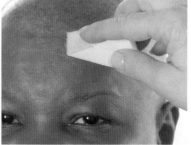

- Good light is a must. Fluorescent lighting, found in most stores, can alter color. Either take a small color sample home, or apply some to your forehead and walk out into the daylight to check color.

- Your skin may be a different shade right now. If you appear more gray, that doesn't mean you should pick out a gray foundation! For most skin tones, foundations that have yellow undertones work well by warming up the skin for a natural look. They provide a more balanced base than foundations containing red or orange undertones. Those really do make the skin look red or orange!

- If you think you need a slightly lighter or darker shade than the one you are using, try mixing foundations together in a small bottle to create a more suitable color.

Techniques

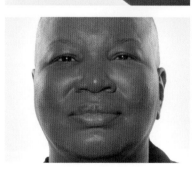

- Apply foundation either with your finger or a sponge. (Sponges tend to retain product, resulting in a lighter application to your face. Using your finger can give you better control.)

- Dab foundation on your forehead, on the top of your nose, above your lip, and on your chin. Make three triangle dots on your cheeks and blend. Always blend across your forehead, making even, long strokes. Start out with a light application. You can always add more.

- Wherever you've applied camouflage, apply your foundation gently over the area with a press-pat motion. Be careful not to rub or pull the skin.

- Make long downward strokes to the face, stopping at the jawline and rolling under the jaw to blend. Don't apply foundation to your neck or you'll end up with nowhere to stop. You certainly don't want to go from your forehead to your toes!

- For a light pick-me-up, apply foundation only on areas that really call for it. By press-patting foundation on these spots you will blend it right in.

Once you've finished applying your foundation, you will have created a polished appearance for your face and protected your skin from wind, sun, and other harsh conditions.

Under-Eye Concealer

Under-Eye Concealer and
Highlighter

Texture and Color

Application

Points to Remember

"The difference in the way my eyes look before and after — it's amazing!"

— Elizabeth Q.

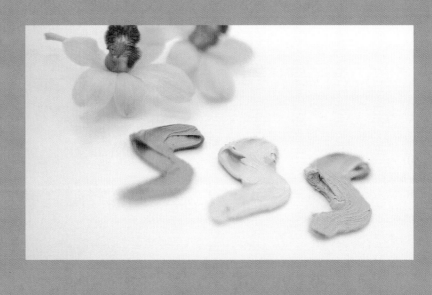

Under-Eye Concealer

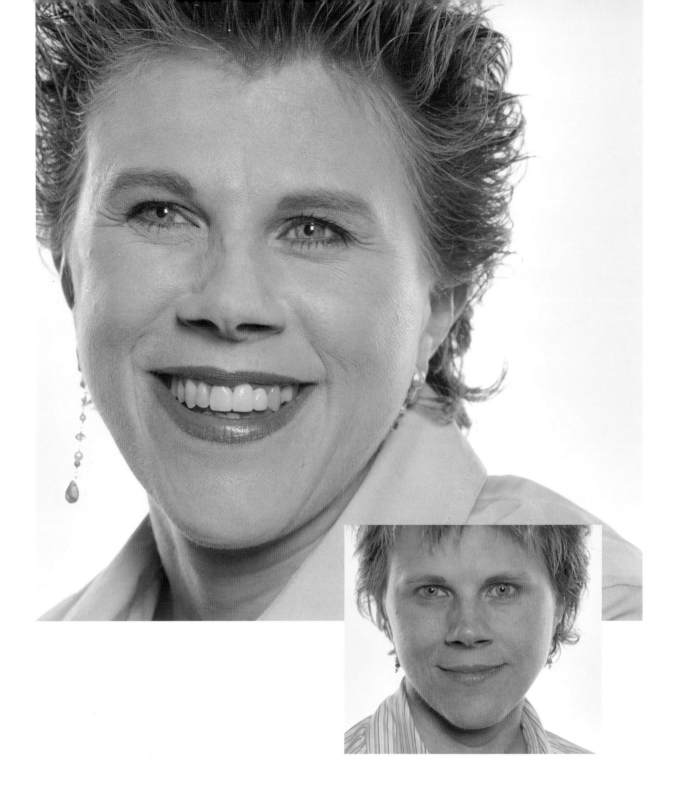

"Wow! I can't believe the difference! I can finally get rid of the darkness underneath my eyes. The trick is so easy, even I can do it!"

– Jennifer F.

UNDER-EYE CONCEALER AND HIGHLIGHTER

The technique I use to apply under-eye concealer is a unique method. This technique not only covers up dark circles under your eyes but also enhances and perks up the entire eye area. Everything with makeup is highlight and shadow, and under-eye concealer is one of the most effective tools to create the illusion that highlight and shadow provide.

Every person who has tried this technique is amazed! Step back from the mirror, observe the difference after you've used the technique on one eye, and notice the big change before and after concealer.

Note: This technique for under-eye concealer is used on top of foundation.

If you were going in order of putting on makeup, you'd do the following: skin care, camouflage, foundation. Then under-eye concealer. If you are not using foundation, just apply concealer after camouflage.

Texture and Color

Concealer is sold in pots, wands, and sticks. When choosing a color, concealer should be one shade lighter than your foundation, or your skin tone if you're not using foundation. The texture should not be too thick or it will emphasize any lines around the eyes.

If you have foundation one shade lighter than you are now using, that can serve as your concealer.

Application

- Use a concealer brush or wand.

- Draw a line with the brush down the side of your nose, starting at the tear duct area and extending down to the nostril.

- Draw an arc under your eye from the inner corner to slightly past the outer corner.

- Connect the line from the bottom of your nostril up to meet the other line where it stopped slightly outside the eyebrow.

- Notice the sideways triangle pattern you've just created. The most important part of the application is that you stay in this area.

- Take a small amount of the concealer on your finger and put it in the triangle area – just a little bit.

- Press-pat gently and remove the excess from your finger with a tissue. Press-pat the product all over the area. Touch down lightly, and pat it to move the product along. *Stay in the triangle area.* It's a must!

- Look straight into the mirror. Make sure the concealer is well-blended and the line of demarcation you used to create the triangle is gone. By press-patting on the line until it's well-blended it will seem to disappear.

Compare the eye you've just made up to your other eye. You'll be absolutely amazed at the difference! See how much brighter the eye looks? This technique is also flattering because it gives the illusion of a stronger cheekbone and brightens the whole face.

Points to Remember

- Do not rub or pull at the skin. Just press-pat.

- You should not be able to see where the color stops and starts.

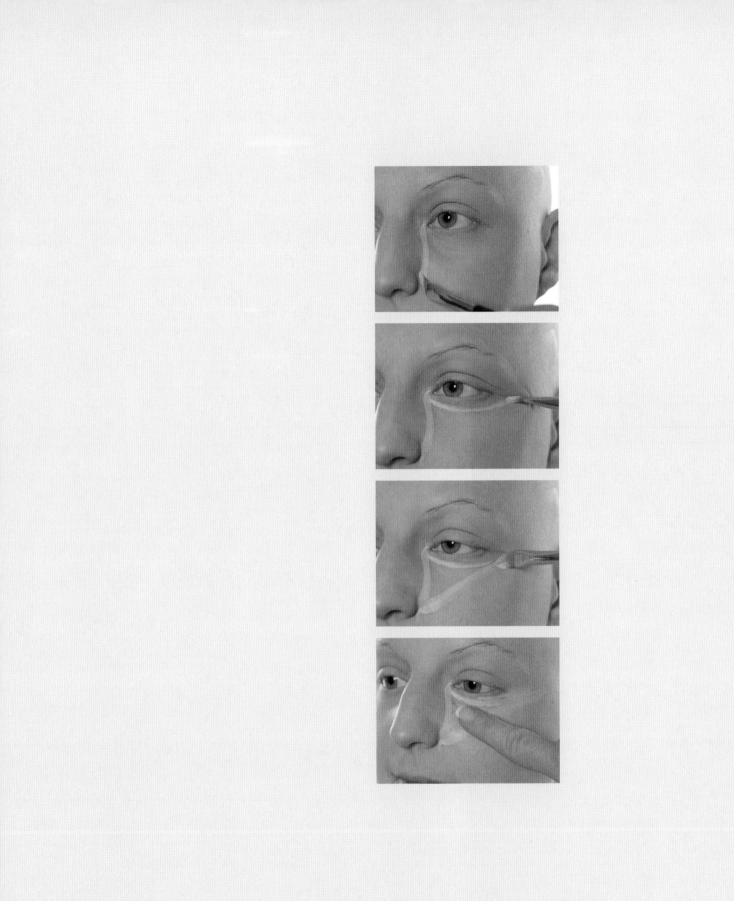

Under-Eye Concealer

"This is all part

a surviv

– *Matthew A.*

of being
vor."

Under-Eye Concealer

Powder 7

Introduction to Powder

Types of Powders

Selecting the Right Color
and Texture

Effective Techniques for
Applying Powder

"Makeup gave me the courage to get out of bed in the morning."

— Pamela R.

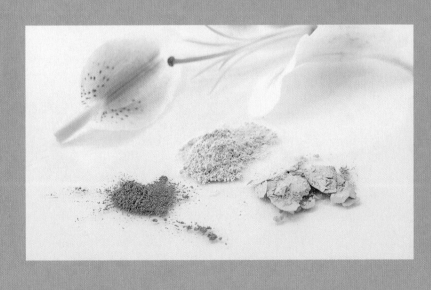

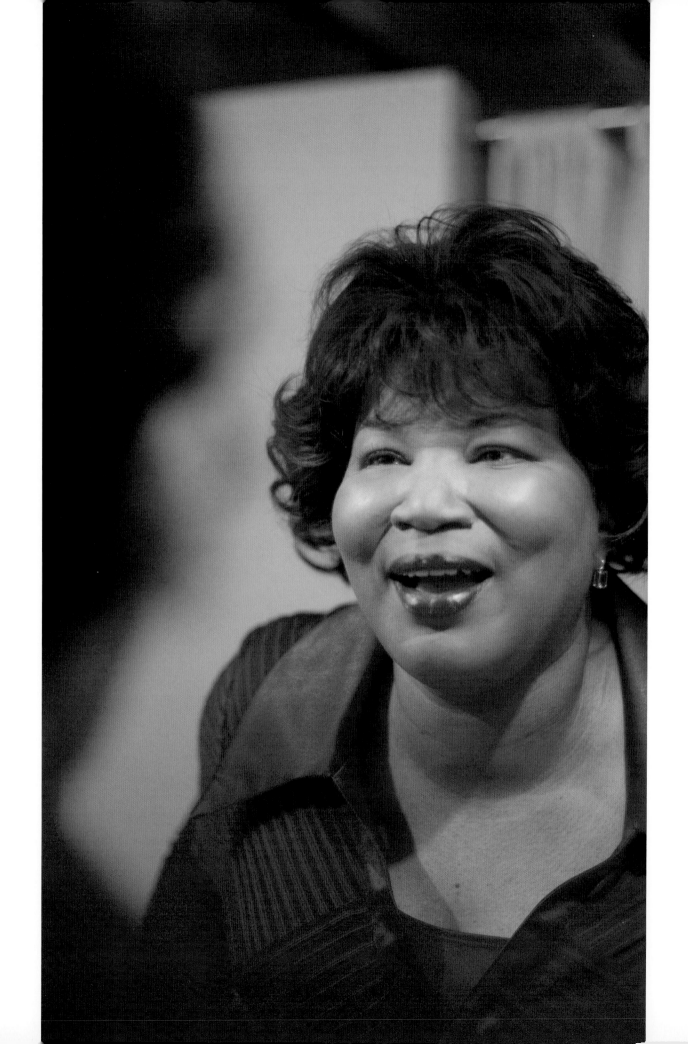

POWDER

Powder is used to set foundation and concealer and absorb natural facial oils. Even when worn alone, powder prevents an oily shine from forming. As you create your natural look and cover up imperfections, the addition of powder gives your complexion a clean, polished look. Try carrying a small pressed-powder compact with you so you can do touch-ups and maintain your makeup throughout the day.

Types of Powder

- Loose powder: a very fine-grained powder, applied with a large brush. The finer the grain of powder the more natural the outcome. This is a stay-at-home powder. If you carry it with you, it can easily spill and create a mess!

- Pressed powder: a very fine quality of powder in compact form, used with a powder puff or sponge. By applying it in a press-pat motion, you end up with a very polished look. Great for on-the-go application!

- Dual-action powder: a wet/dry formula that comes in a compact. This type of powder leaves a high-quality matte finish with opaque coverage. Used wet and applied with a dampened sponge, it can be worn as foundation. If used dry, apply it with a sponge or brush over foundation.

- Translucent powder: Not recommended! Tends to look chalky and artificial on most skin colors.

- Luxury powder: This is a more "high-tech" powder that deflects unflattering light and gives an especially smooth finish.

- Powder papers: These are small in size but big on delivery. Not only are they effective in blotting excess oils and touching up makeup, they're easy to carry around, too!

Color and Texture

- For loose or pressed powder, select shades that have yellow undertones. As with foundation, these shades will look most flattering and natural.

- Yellow tones distract from any redness and lighten up dark circles and imperfections.

- Not all powders are created equal – look for ones that feel smooth and silky to the touch, and that are invisible on the skin.

- Dual-finish powders should match your foundation color exactly.

Technique

- Apply loose or pressed powder with a powder puff. Press-pat onto the skin, followed by dusting off the excess with a big soft brush.

- To polish your complexion and look the most natural, go across the forehead and then make quick downward strokes on the rest of your face.

Common Mistakes With Powder

Looking too white. Powder shouldn't make you look like a ghost. If you appear too white, then your product is too light. Try selecting a shade with a more yellow tone.

Ending up with skin that's too dry and makeup that's too cakey. The most likely problem is too much powder. Lighten up on the amount of powder and use a large brush to distribute the powder evenly on your face. If your foundation is too drying, you may need to add more moisture to the skin.

Using a powder with a strong fragrance. Avoid this type of powder. Don't risk sensitivity to the fragrance.

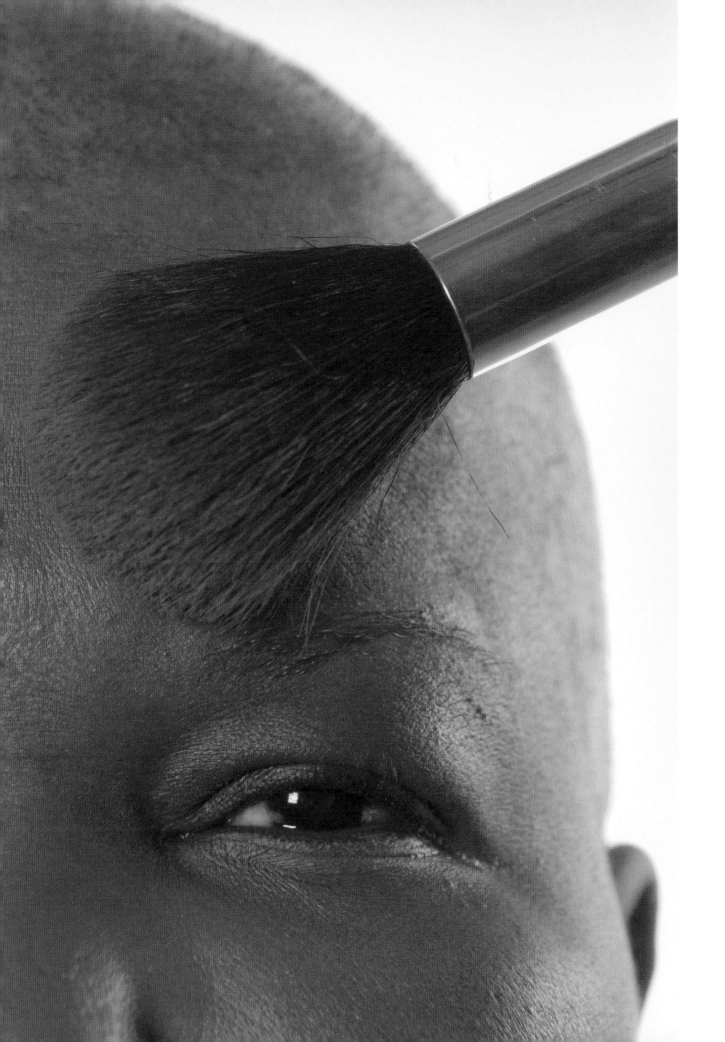

Eyebrows

"It was more traumatic for me to lose my eyebrow
hair than the hair on my head."

— Marie R.

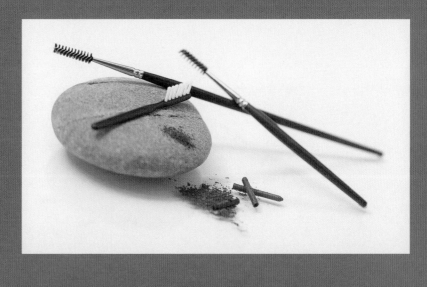

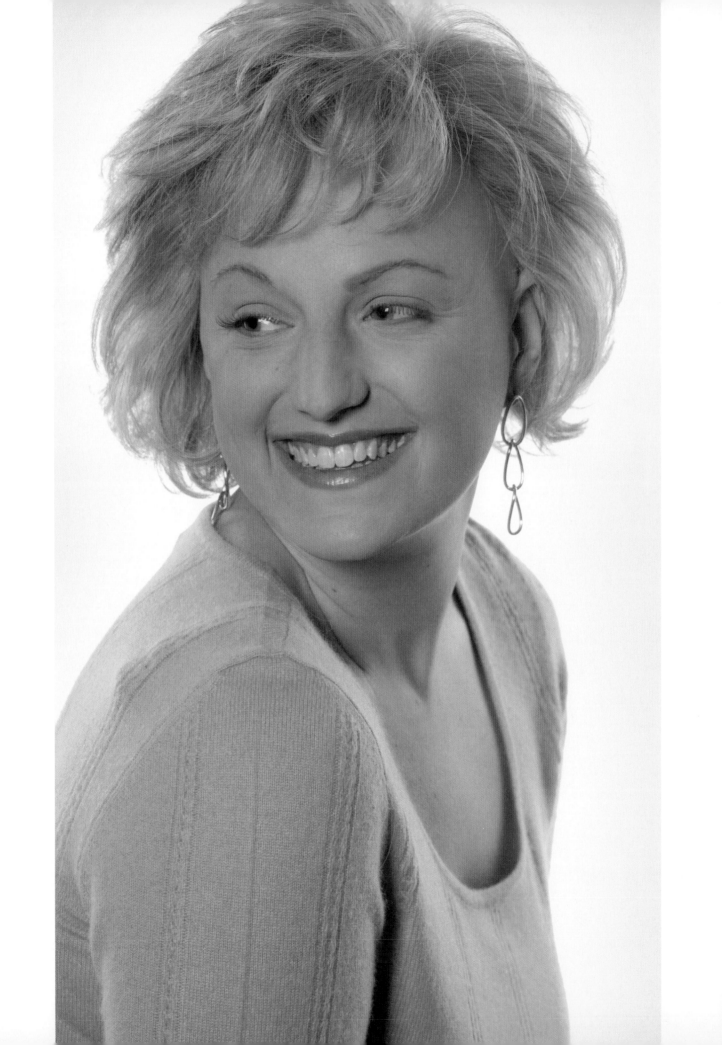

EYEBROWS

This is the best time to do your eyebrows. By doing them now, you add color and balance, and you can clearly see your whole face coming together. There's a sense of instant gratification when you see your eyebrow line has formed. The eyebrows are such a big part of the complete lesson!

The eyebrows are a very prominent feature on the face. Thick, thin, shapely, or natural, the brows reflect a very personal style. For many, the loss of eyebrows is a tough challenge, no matter whether you've lost your brows or they're noticeably thinning. Approach your brows in a different way than you have before, especially if you never really knew how to groom them well. These techniques provide a clear, comprehensive way, at every stage of the growth or loss of eyebrow hair, to achieve brows that look natural – not drawn-on!

"I hear a sigh of relief when I tell people 'Yes! You can *create natural-looking eyebrows.'"*

– Lori Ovitz

Tools

This is what you need to do your eyebrows properly, whether you have no hair at all, partial hair, or full brows.

Pencil: For making eyebrows, you need to have a fine stroke. It's best to use a pencil that's hard and thin. Thick pencils make it harder to control the size of your strokes, and soft pencils tend to smudge. Note: If your pencil is too soft, or softens as you use it, you can put it in the refrigerator to harden.

Powder or eye shadow: These are basically the same product with the same consistency, just different packaging. If you have eye shadow at home, you don't have to run out to buy eyebrow powder. In fact, a nice eye shadow works just great, as long as it has a matte finish. Eye shadow that is shiny or frosted does not work for brows.

Brush: This is a flat, stiff, hard-angled brush designed specifically for eyebrows.

Grooming tool: Any small brush or comb that enables you to brush through your finished brows is fine. For example, you can use an old, cleaned mascara brush or even a disinfected toothbrush.

Sealer: This is a clear gel that's the finishing touch to fix your eyebrows. You can buy a product that's specifically called an eyebrow sealer. Or you can just use clear mascara. Some people even use hair spray. I don't recommend it because it can irritate your skin, and it can flake off. In a pinch, however, it can be an option.

Accessories

Cotton swabs can be a great help in cleaning up stray marks.

Small scissors: Often called manicure scissors, these are small scissors with rounded tips. They are great for snipping off eyebrows hairs that are too long.

Tweezers: For plucking eyebrow hairs, I recommend tweezers with a slanted edge and a tight grip.

Choosing Colors

The objective in makeup application is to achieve a look that is natural. Choosing the best color for you is a big part of this process. For eyebrows, there are two items that involve color: eyebrow pencil, and eyebrow powder/eye shadow.

To get that natural look, choose a color one shade lighter than your hair color. There's an exception: If you have blond or very light hair, don't go a shade lighter.

I have found that shades ranging from taupe to light brown work best for most people, unless their hair is very dark. An important consideration: You don't want your eyebrow color to overpower your eyes. Following are my color recommendations for eyebrow pencil and powder based on hair color:

HAIR COLOR	EYEBROW SHADE
blond, strawberry blond, light brown	taupe or light brown
auburn	taupe or light brown
medium brown hair	taupe or light brown
dark brown hair	dark brown
black	dark brown *(may be mixed with a little black if result is too brown)*
dark black	soft black *(may mix with brown to warm it up)*

"Take bac

k control."

— *Rachael M.*

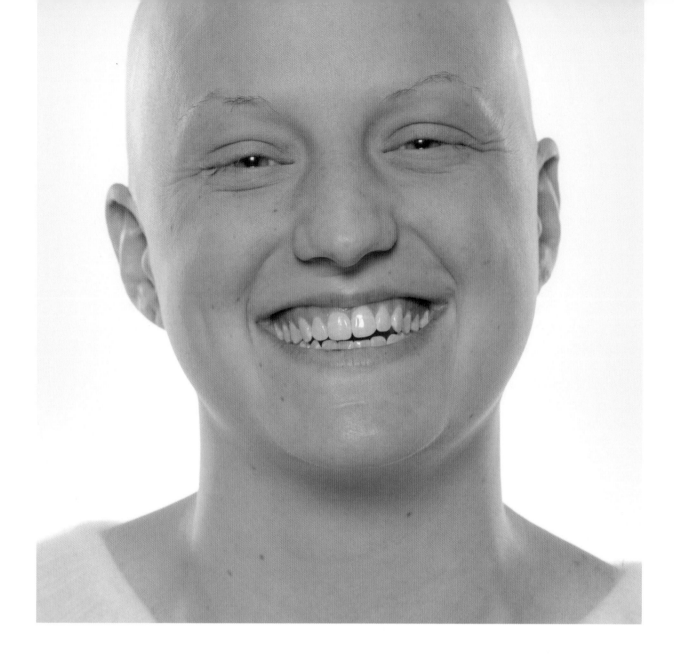

Creating Eyebrows

There are three different scenarios in designing eyebrows:

1. You have no hair on your brows at all.

2. You have partial hair loss or hair regrowth.

3. You have a full brow.

While I am going to focus first on building eyebrows when you have no hair at all, the techniques also apply to eyebrows with partial or full hair. In later sections of this chapter, you'll find information on tweezing and finishing up eyebrows with hair.

Identifying the Flow Line of the Eyebrow

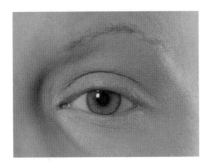

STEP 1: FINDING THE EYEBROW BONE

The easiest way to decide where to put your eyebrow is to feel it. I have put makeup on thousands of faces, and I can tell you this with certainty: With every person's facial structure, you can actually feel what shape the natural eyebrow line wants to be and where it wants to go. It's called the eyebrow bone.

You may never have specifically noticed this bone before or tried to find it. Even without a wisp of hair, however, you can identify it. Your eyebrow goes directly on this natural line – not above it or below it, but right smack on it. Here's how to find it:

• Look straight into the mirror.

• Take your finger and place it above your eye.

• Now run your finger along the bone that protrudes above the eye.

• Start at any point and just let your finger move back and forth.

• Although there is a lot of bone in that area, your finger will automatically ride along the natural protrusion of bone that ordinarily lies directly underneath the eyebrow.

• By doing this exercise, you have identified the line where your brow belongs.

STEP 2: DEFINING THE DOTS – WHERE YOUR EYEBROW STARTS, ARCHES, AND ENDS

Every eyebrow has a starting point, a natural arch, and an ending point. There's a way to find just where each of these should be placed, even without any hair at all to guide you. You start by defining three key dots, and then you fill in the areas between those dots.

Starting Point

- Use your eyebrow pencil. (Note: You can use the handle of your eyebrow brush instead. Whatever you use – even a regular pencil is okay – the length of the shaft must be at least four inches long.)

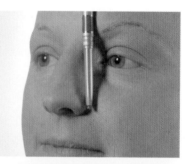

- Put the lower end of the pencil alongside the lower part of your nostril where it flares out.

- Put the upper end of the pencil straight up from the nostril alongside the inner corner of your eye.

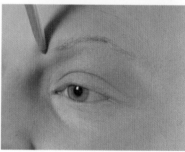

- Make a dot where the upper end of the pencil meets the brow line you've already identified in Step 1.

- You have identified where your eyebrow should start.

Ending Point

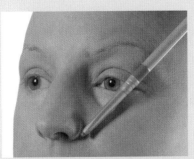

- Once again, put the lower end of the eyebrow pencil alongside your lower nostril where it flares out.

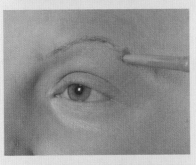

- This time, angle the upper end of the pencil so that it reaches the outer corner of your eye.

- Make a dot where the upper end of the pencil meets the brow line you've already identified.

- You have identified where your eyebrow should end.

Natural, Upward Curve

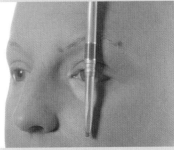

- Take your eyebrow pencil again.

- Hold the pencil straight in front of the iris of your eye (the black middle of the eye).

- Make a third dot at the spot where the pencil meets the brow line defined by the dots in the first two steps.

- You have identified where your eyebrow should arch.

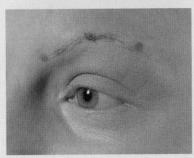

With these three dots, you have lined up your eyebrow – where to start, where to stop, and where the arch should be located.

Creating Natural-Looking Eyebrows Without Any Hair or With Partial Hair/Hair Regrowth

STEP 1: THE EYEBROW PENCIL – CREATING HAIR-LIKE STROKES

The secret is in the stroke – light and feathery. This is the stroke you use to apply both pencil and powder in the spaces between the three dots that define the length and shape of the brow. The result is a brow that replicates natural hair.

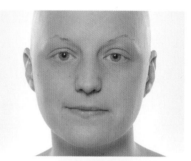

As you go through the following steps, keep in mind that an eyebrow generally has a thicker part at the beginning, a middle part that arches up slightly, and an end that thins out. Think of the eyebrow not as a line, but a flow.

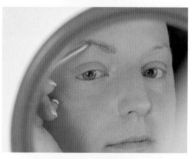

- Feel the eyebrow pencil in your hand. Resist the temptation to press hard or make thick, heavy marks.

- Place your pencil at the starting point you've already identified – right on the dot.

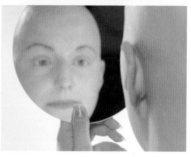

- Hold the pencil at a slight angle, poised to make a small stroke that goes from the bottom to the top.

- Now begin to make very soft strokes – light, feathery, hair-like.

- Imagine yourself making little hairs – one at a time. If you find that you are having difficulty applying color with your pencil, try this technique: Make a fist. Rub the pencil point on your hand in the area between the thumb and the fingers. This "warms up" the pencil and makes the color easier to apply.

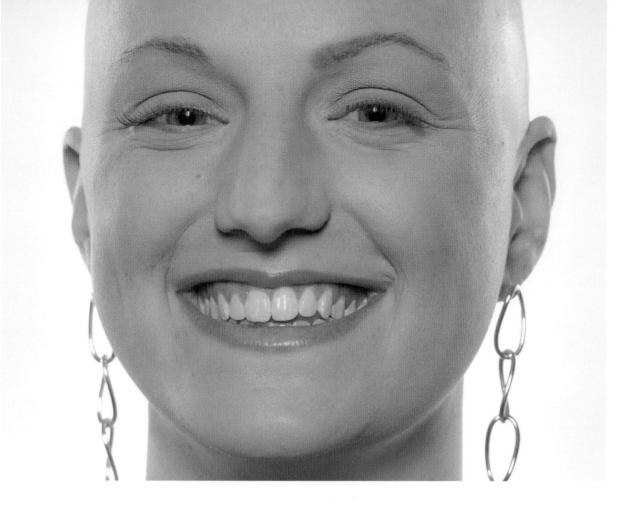

- As you make strokes, connect the dots, going from the first dot to the one that defines the arch. When you approach the dot at the arch, shorten and raise the strokes, slanting upward.

- Make fewer strokes at the arch, and then continue to taper the number of strokes as you create the end of the eyebrow, which is the thinnest part of the brow.

- If you have a scar on the brow line, use your pencil to make dots on the scar, applying more pressure than you do with the feathery motion of the hair-like strokes.

Now, assess what you've done. Have you gone out of the eyebrow area? Made strokes that are too thick? Angled lines in the opposite direction? Not to worry. The beauty of makeup is that you can easily change it. Take a cotton swab and gently wipe off any strokes that don't look right.

As you can see from these guidelines, you are *not* going to draw a line from one end of your eye to the other. Instead, you are going to mimic natural hair using light, feathery strokes.

After you have completed one eyebrow, go on to the other. At the end of your efforts, you will have two natural-looking eyebrows, right on top of the brow bone, formed by little hair-like strokes at an angle.

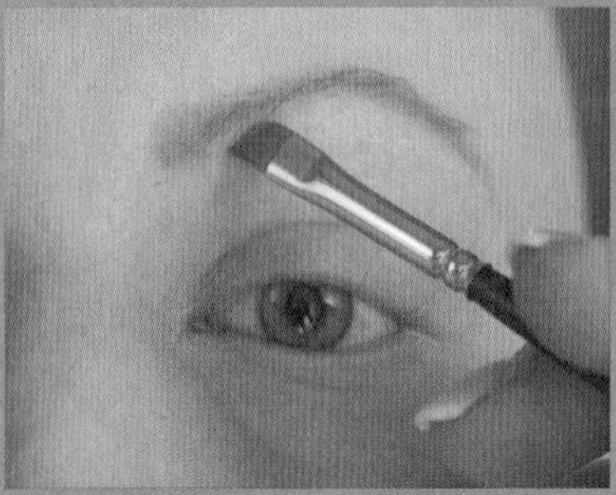
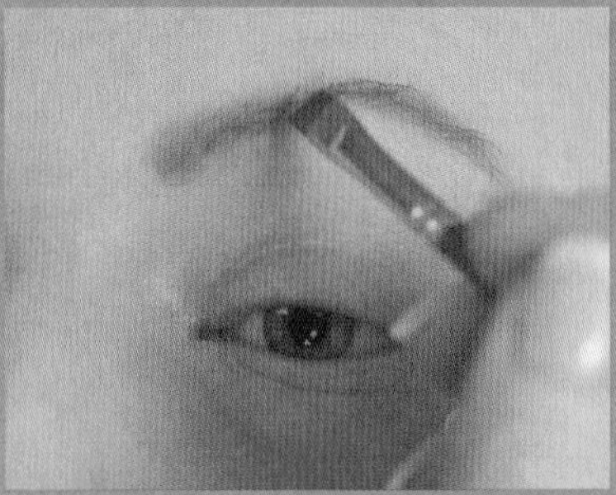
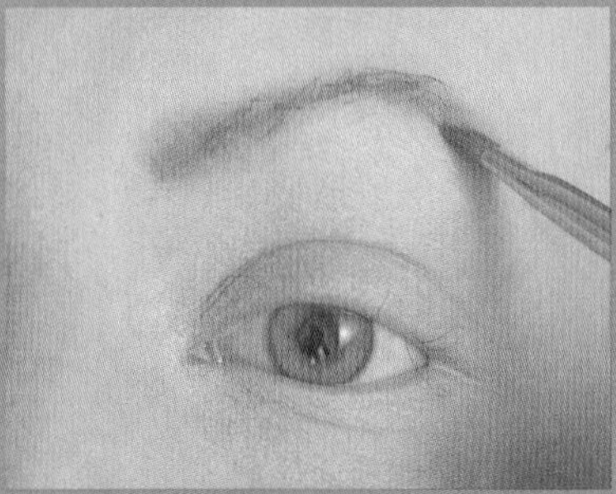

STEP 2: EYEBROW POWDER (OR EYE SHADOW AS POWDER): CREATING DEPTH AND DENSITY

With Step 1, you've come a long way in forming a pair of eyebrows. But you're not done yet! Now you will add powder strokes to your pencil work to create both depth and density in your brows. This combination really makes the brow come together. It creates a natural look since eyebrow powder gives the pencil strokes more texture, making them look more like hair.

A further benefit is that the powder helps the newly created brow stay on better. You don't have to worry about your eyebrow "melting." Powder locks in the pencil, and you can expect the brow to stay on until you wash it off.

- Use your eyebrow brush. It should have a small, angled edge with hard bristles that gradually get longer.

- Put the brush into the eye shadow or eyebrow powder.

- Tap off the extra powder.

- Using the powdered angled edge, go over the strokes you made with the pencil. If you covered a scar with dots, put powder over that area too.

- Notice how the pencil strokes combine with the powder to add more depth and definition to the eyebrow.

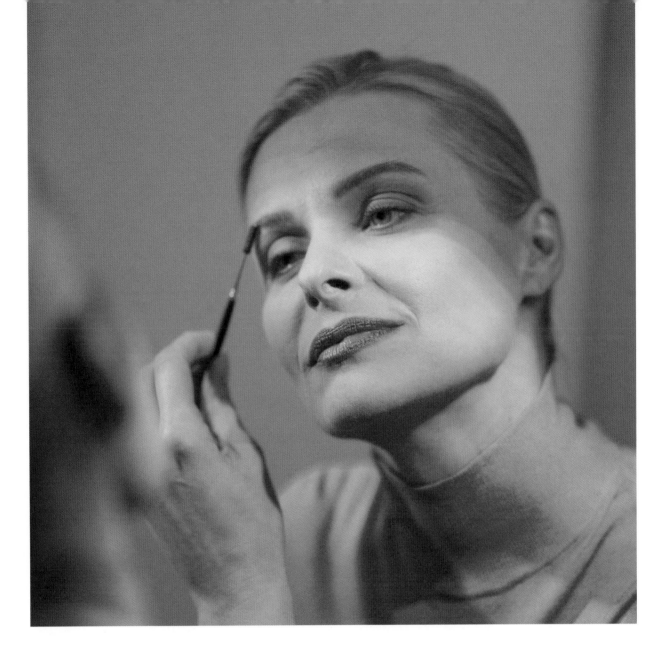

- If you have difficulty applying the color, or if the color is too dark, use your hand as a palette. Make a fist, and apply the powder to the area between your thumb and fingers. Then take your eyebrow brush and gently rub it back and forth over the color on your hand. Now, apply the color from your brush to your eyebrow. This results in a softer color.

- After you've finished applying color, use your eyebrow grooming brush, which can be a mascara brush, toothbrush, or other small-bristled brush.

- Brush upward along the eyebrow you've been creating, going from bottom to top, in the direction that hairs would naturally grow.

- Continue brushing to combine the pencil strokes with the powder strokes.

STEP 3: EYEBROW SEALER – THE FINISHING TOUCH

You're ready to seal in your strokes!

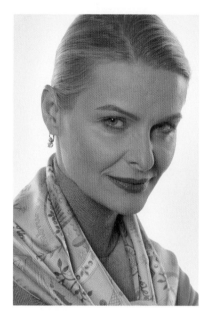

- Take the brush from your eyebrow sealer or clear mascara and dip it into the gel. You only need a little bit.

- Brush the sealer over the eyebrows.

- Now sit back and take a good look at what you've created!

You'll be amazed again and again with the finished product. Don't be discouraged if it's not perfect the first time. It takes practice to master the technique. And if you see something you don't like, keep those cotton swabs handy. You can use them to wipe away any stray marks.

Once you've followed the directions outlined in Steps 1, 2, and 3, you can experience how it's entirely possible – with minimal supplies, a set of instructions, and a dose of patience – to create natural-looking eyebrows where no eyebrows existed before. In fact, I've worked with many people with either no brows or partial brows who've said that even their natural brows never looked so good!

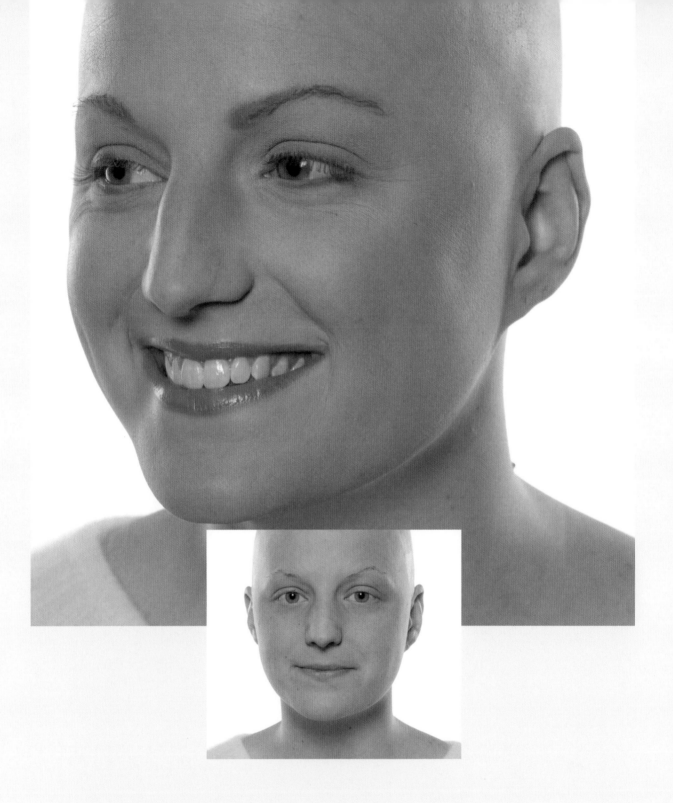

*"My eyebrows look better than ever! I finally learned how to do
them correctly — and create a natural look!"*

— Martha F.

Partial Hair Loss and Hair Regrowth

You may not lose all your eyebrow hair during treatment, or you may be at the point in your treatment when your hair is starting to grow back. Instead of a bare brow, you may be dealing with half a brow, or a brow that is spotted with hair. Don't be discouraged by the uneven look. Rather, you can use that hair as the basis for building a full, more attractive brow.

The initial steps are the same as building a brow from scratch. The difference is that now you treat stray hairs as you would if you were grooming an eyebrow with full hair – tweeze, trim, and clean up.

- Choose an eyebrow pencil and eyebrow powder or eye shadow in a color that is most like the color of your existing brow hair.

- Follow the steps in the section on Identifying the Flow Line of the Eyebrow. Review how to line up the beginning point, the arch, and the end of your eyebrow.

- Wherever hair is lacking along the eyebrow, fill in those areas with the same light, feathery strokes identified in the section on Creating Natural-Looking Eyebrows. Make feathery pencil strokes in bare areas on the brow or where the hair is too thin. Then apply powder over the entire brow to create uniform depth and density.

- As you work on your eyebrow, notice any stray or out-of-place hairs. Eliminate them by tweezing. For tips on techniques for tweezing and treating eyebrow hair, see the following section on Grooming Full Eyebrows.

- Finish with your eyebrow grooming brush to gently brush the brow in place, using a motion that is angled upward.

- When you are satisfied with the look you've created, apply eyebrow sealer or clear mascara to keep the eyebrow in place.

- Repeat these steps on your other eyebrow.

Grooming Full Eyebrows

Perhaps you did not lose eyebrow hair during treatment, or your treatments are completed and your hair has grown back. Instead of asking, "How do I create natural-looking eyebrows when there are only partial hairs or none at all?", you have a different question: "How can my eyebrows now look the best possible?"

The following are key points in creating beautiful brows for now and in the future:

WAXING

I'm not a fan of waxing eyebrows, especially for people undergoing chemotherapy or radiation. The skin is much too sensitive at this time, and waxing can be painful. But at any time, waxing has its drawbacks. Sure, it keeps unwanted hairs away for a longer period of time. But it's far too easy to make a mistake while waxing. In my experience, I've often needed to go back and tweeze even after a good waxing.

DYES AND LIGHTENING CREAMS

If you are considering using these products, be sure to check with your doctor first. I don't recommend using dyes or lightening creams that could affect your skin while you are using medications or having treatments.

TWEEZING TIPS

When it's obvious that some hairs are not part of your eyebrow shape, tweeze them out. These are typically ones that are under your brow or between your eyes.

The best time to groom and tweeze the eyebrows is right after a shower. The pores are open, and it's much easier and less painful to pluck the hairs out. Grab each hair you want to remove, one at a time, and pluck from the root of the hair in the direction it grows. Plucking from the root helps stop breakage of the hair and prevents the hair from growing back quickly.

Some people find it helpful to gently pull the skin taut with the opposite hand while plucking. Remember never to pull too hard on the eye area because it is very delicate. Whatever tweezing technique works for you, make sure of two things: that your hands are clean and your tweezers are disinfected.

PAIN WHEN TWEEZING

I believe in good tools. If you have the proper tweezers, you should be able to substantially reduce discomfort. If you experience discomfort, or find little red bumps on your skin after you tweeze, try applying a cold compress on top of the sore spots.

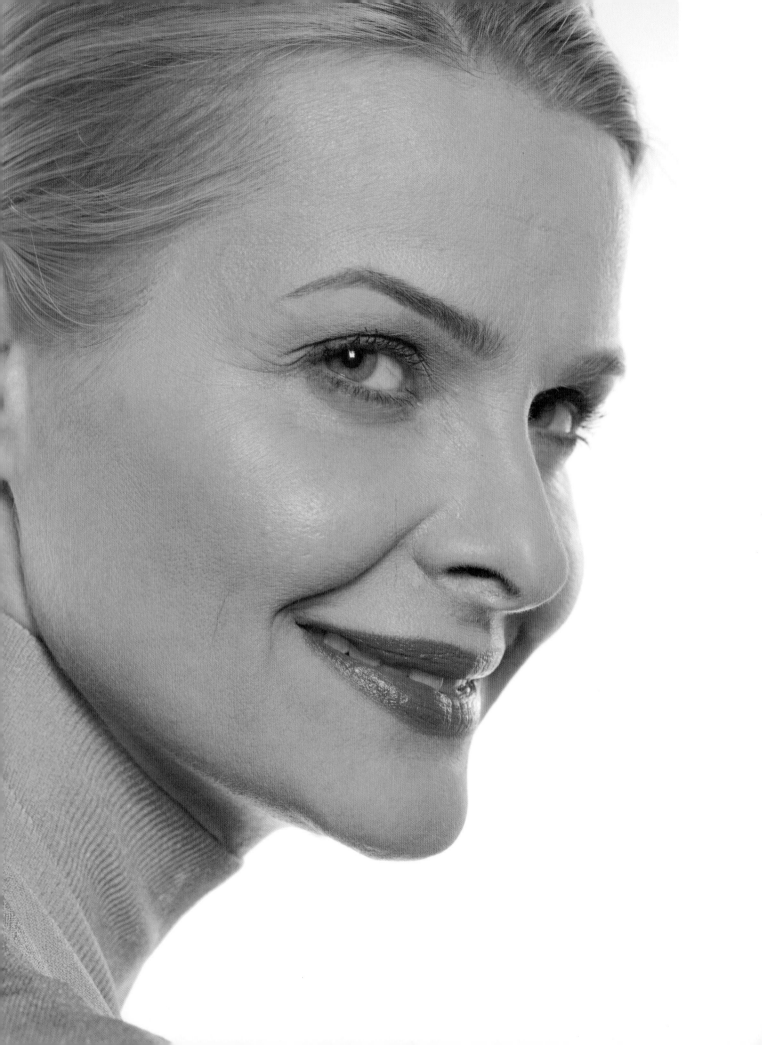

TRIMMING EYEBROWS – JUST A SNIP WILL DO THE TRICK

Many people wonder if they can trim eyebrow hairs that are too long. Absolutely! First brush your eyebrows in an upward direction. Notice any long hairs that curl out. Then cut them with a pair of manicure scissors. If you don't have manicure scissors, use any pair of short scissors with a rounded tip. Short scissors will give you better control, and rounded tips prevent punctures.

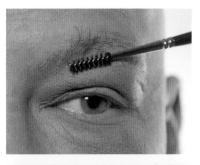

Cut eyebrow hairs at an angle. Your eyebrow hairs grow on a slant, so they should also be cut on a slant. Angle the scissors in your hand so that the cut is done in the same direction as your eyebrows grow. Then brush the brow back in place. Trimming hairs with a well-placed snip really makes a difference in the shape of the brows.

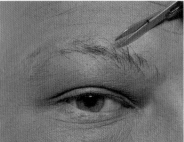

ACHIEVING A CLEAN, FINISHED LOOK

Looking straight in the mirror, study your eyebrow. Make adjustments to any stray hairs on that natural line by tweezing and snipping. If you're not sure where the boundaries of your eyebrow should be, review the section on Identifying the Flow Line of the Eyebrow.

Check underneath your brows. Are there stray hairs? If so, lift up the look of your brows by tweezing.

Now look on top of your brows. There used to be a myth that it was against the rules to tweeze on top of the eyebrows. Nonsense! There are no official rules. The only guideline is to create a look that is best for you. And if there are stray hairs at the top of the eyebrow, they can create a shadow effect and make your eyebrow line look incomplete and somewhat messy. They can even make you look like you're angry or scowling. What to do about the hair that appears on the top of an otherwise well-defined brow line? Pluck, pluck, pluck.

If you really have trouble creating the look you want, I suggest you consider going to a makeup professional who can define the shape of your brows. Just one trip to a talented expert should help you be clear about the flow of your brows and enable you to maintain them yourself. This can be especially helpful if you are having difficulty establishing the arch of your brow.

EYEBROWS THAT GROW DOWNWARD AT THE END

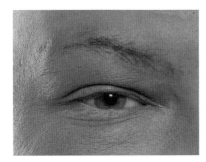

Take out the hairs that are slouching. A downward drift at the end can really make your hair and eyes look more droopy and sad. Makeup is working with illusion. What you are creating with your brows is a face that's perked up, picked up, and refreshed. After you tweeze the end hair, establish a new, brighter look with your pencil and powder strokes.

EYEBROWS THAT ARE TOO LIGHT

Try adding a light dusting of eyebrow powder in a shade darker than your natural eyebrow color. This works wonders in perking up and showing off light eyebrows.

LOOKING LIKE A PHOTOGRAPH

Stop trying! Eyebrows are not a fashion statement; they are a reflection of the best features of your own face. Eyebrows are there to frame *your* eyes, not somebody else's. So what if super-thin is in? Don't torture yourself trying to pluck so many hairs that your eyebrow hurts a lot, won't flow properly, and doesn't look good on your face! Your objective is to create well-groomed, clean eyebrows that fit your basic eye shape and follow a pattern that flows naturally on your face.

MATCHING BOTH EYEBROWS

The best way to do this is practice. If you follow the guidelines discussed in this chapter, you'll be pleased at how both brows will match.

Conclusion

Whether you've created eyebrows from scratch, added to partial brows, or improved existing brows, all you have to do now is look in the mirror and enjoy the fruits of your efforts. And always keep in mind that, thanks to using the power of makeup wisely applied, you are restoring your own natural features that have been temporarily altered.

Notice how the eyebrows provide a frame to your eyes. See how cleaned-up, finished eyebrows, with natural hair or without, have given a huge lift to your face. Congratulate yourself on how you've used a little eye geometry by skillfully angling a pencil on the flow line. Appreciate how you've combined the simple strokes of pencil and powder with an appropriate choice of color to make a realistic brow. Remember, for now or for the future, that snips and plucks can bring unruly hairs into line. And don't forget to practice. It gets easier and quicker the more you do it.

Take time to enjoy the look of your new eyebrows in the privacy of your own mirror and in your public encounters. You can be confident that you are doing precisely what you need to do – using makeup as a tool to help you look your best!

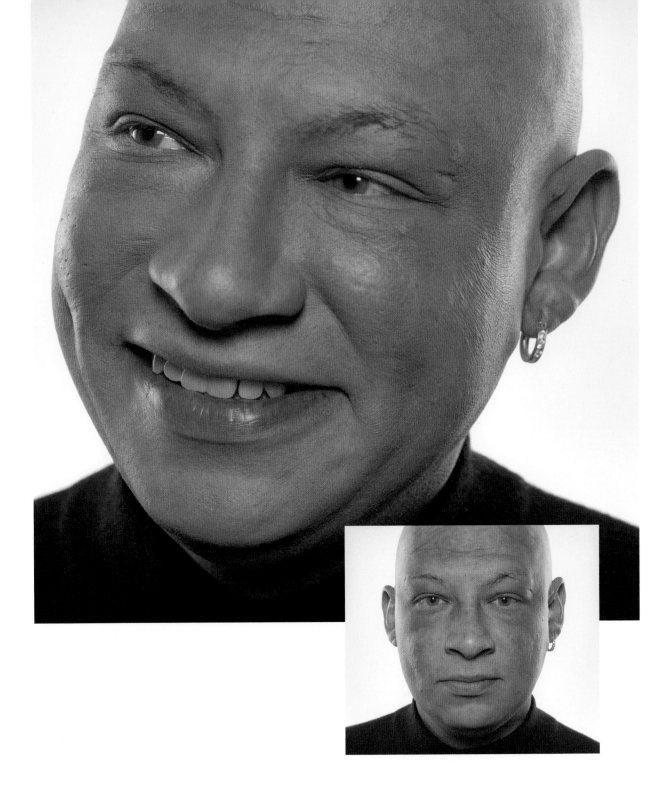

"Having gone through what I have, I want to tell all cancer patients that there is a rainbow at the end of all this treatment – the rainbow of life."

– Angel L. Colon, Jr.

Eyebrows

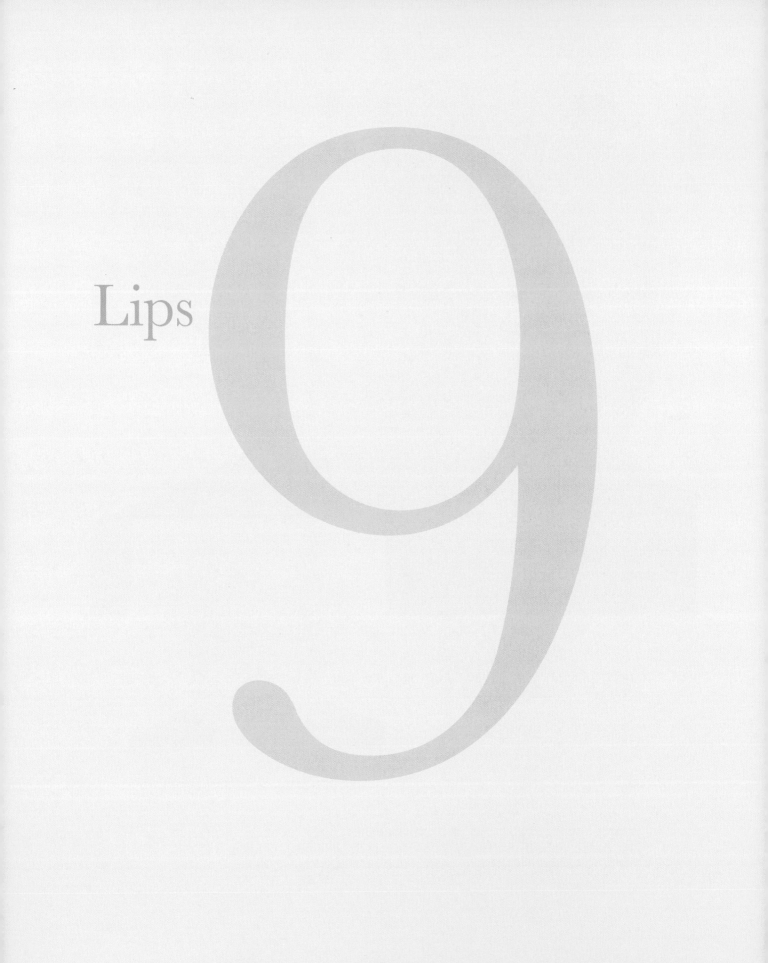

Lips

9

"You mean there's a way to keep my lipstick on for more than an hour?"

– Heather A.

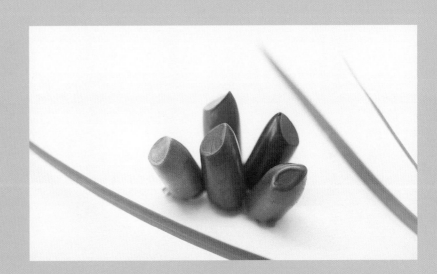

"I'm shocked at the difference just
changing my lipstick made!"

– *Shellby T.*

LIPS

Experiment. Try a totally new shade, or mix two shades together to create a new color. As silly as it sounds, just a change in lip color can feel like an automatic pick-me-up.

Notes

- Check with your doctor to make sure you don't have a medical reason to avoid any ingredients contained in products for the lips.

- Disinfect your lip brush after each use.

- Don't share any lip-care products as they could carry germs.

The tools and techniques you've used so far have transformed your complexion into a smooth canvas. Now it's time to add color to your lips. This next step really brightens your face and takes the effect of your makeup to a new level.

Lip color provides a base to balance the color and intensity of your makeup. If you want a softer tone on your lips, you can balance that with a stronger color around your eyes – or you can do the reverse. In choosing colors, what you plan to wear is also a key factor. The shade of your lipstick should match well with the colors of your clothing.

Lip Prep

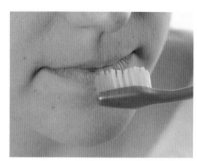

Dry, chapped lips? Try this technique:

- First apply a light amount of lip moisturizing product to the lips.

- Next take a soft toothbrush and lightly stroke the lips to remove the dead skin – also giving your lips a moisturizing treatment!

- If there's any product remaining on your lips, blot it off with a tissue.

Color

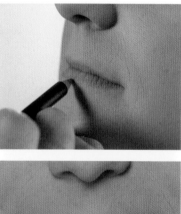

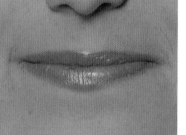

For a quick pick-me-up, simply try a different shade of lipstick. Think about it. If you wear a drab brown lipstick, it's going to make you look drab, too. On the other hand, a more lively color can perk you up. An added benefit of wearing lipstick is that it feels soothing and acts as a coat of protection for your lips.

You can do something as basic as changing the hue of your current lipstick by mixing it with another color that is slightly lighter or darker. Mix several colors together using a bobbin kit or a special compact to put your lipsticks in. Is your lipstick tube getting low? Instead of throwing it away, scrape the remaining lipstick out of the tube with a toothpick and put it into a small container. Then mix it with other colors. It's a great way to prevent waste; there's a lot more color than you think at the bottom of the tube. You also can create new lipstick colors out of the ones you already have by running your lip brush swiftly over your lips, mixing colors together as you go along.

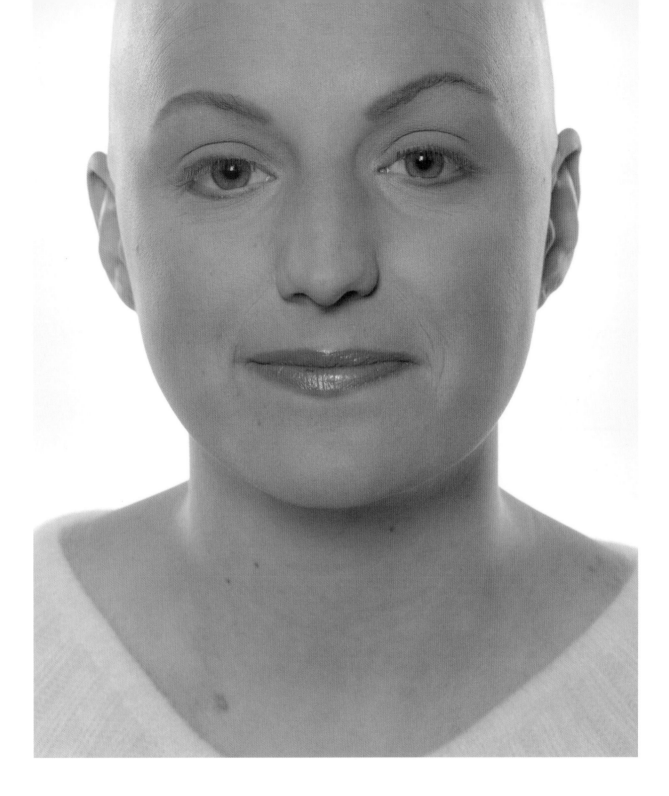

As you can see, there are many options for experimenting with color without purchasing new products. Don't get stuck in a rut.

Choosing Tools for the Lips

Lipstick formulas: What do they mean?

- Sunblock: contains ingredients to protect your lips, typically SPF 15.

- Matte: stays on longest; can be drying.

- Moisture lipstick: just as it says – adds moisture to the lips.

- Stain: very transparent lipstick.

- Frosted: adds glimmer.

- Gloss: wand, pot, or stick form. "Non-gummy" formulas look and feel best. Avoid flavored products.

Lip Pencil

A lip pencil is a corrective tool to even out and enhance the lip shape. It also helps your lipstick stay on longer without smudging.

Selecting the right pencil:

- A thin pencil point is recommended because it gives more control in shaping the lip line.

- A medium-hard pencil works best. A pencil that's too soft is going to melt down and end up running on your lips. A helpful test: Apply a little bit of color on the side of your hand and run your finger over it. If it smudges too easily, it's going to be too soft for the lips.

- The only color you really need is the one that is closest to your natural lip shade.

Lip Liner

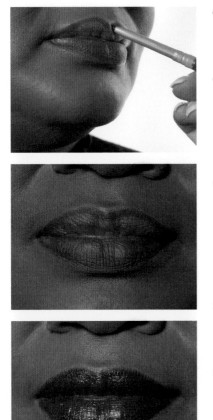

- Looking straight into the mirror, bend your head back with your chin pointing to the mirror.

- A relaxed, closed mouth will enable you to see the natural shape of your lips. Is one side thinner or more pronounced? You can use your lip pencil to smooth out any areas of imbalance.

- Starting in the middle (the bow) of your upper lip, apply right on top of the lip line making corrections as needed. To make lips appear thicker, apply slightly above the natural lip line. To make them appear thinner, apply slightly below the line.

- Use the pencil to draw a line from the middle of the bow to the outer edge. Press gently. Then match the other side.

- Repeat on the bottom: Start in the middle of the lip, go to the outer edge on one side, then match the second side to it.

- Fill in the lips completely with the pencil to help the lipstick stay on and give a more natural-looking lip. After all the lipstick color is gone, you will still have color from the pencil on your lips.

Lipstick

- For more definition and to keep it on longer, apply lipstick with a lip brush.

- If you're trying to cover up a scar, press-pat camouflage on your lip first.

- You can dress up your lipstick by adding lip gloss. (Lip gloss also can be worn alone.)

My Favorite Tricks for Lipstick

- Making lipstick stay on: Take a piece of facial tissue and separate it, making the two-ply into one-ply. Keep your lips together. Hold the tissue in front of you and place it on top of your lips, mouth closed. Take a big powder brush, dip it into some powder, and then press it against your lips. Pull the brush and the tissue away. Go over the area once more with the brush. Now your lipstick will actually stay on all day.

- For a light look: Use lip liner over the entire area and apply lip gloss on top. Gloss adds some color and feels great too.

- Keeping lipstick off your teeth: Take your index finger, open up your lips, put your index finger in your mouth, and close your lips. Pull the index finger out. It's going to get off all the lipstick on the inner portion of your mouth and prevent any of it from getting on your teeth.

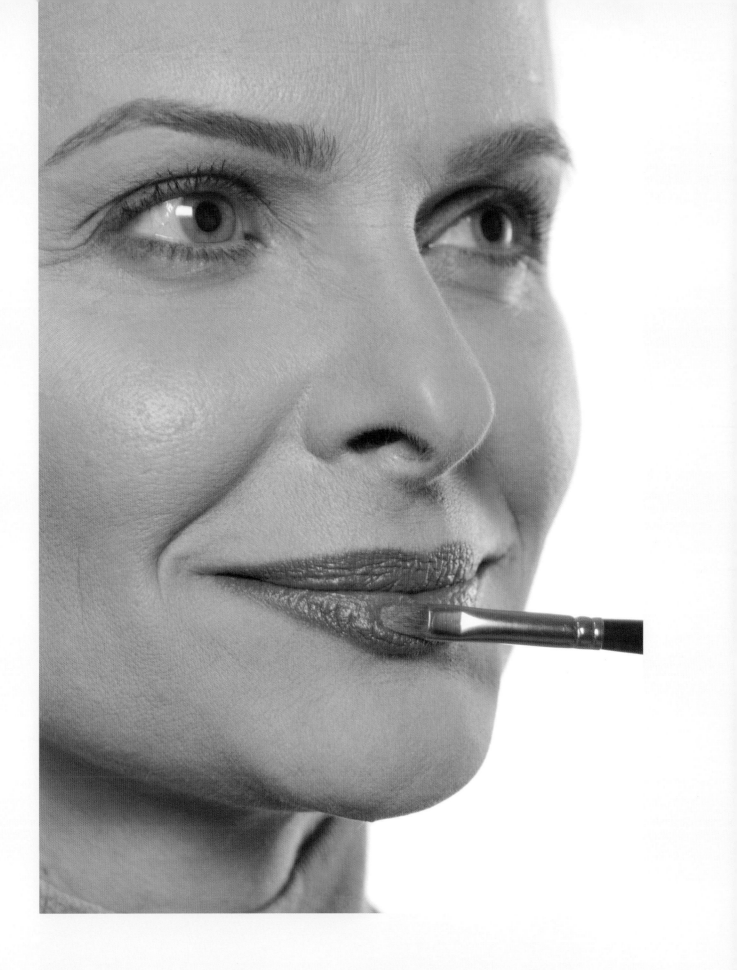

Blush and Bronzer

All About Blush and Bronzer

*"It's not about how you look, it's about who you are inside.
I know that! But I felt so ugly inside too."*

– Rhonda J.

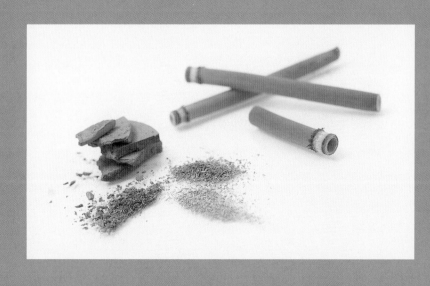

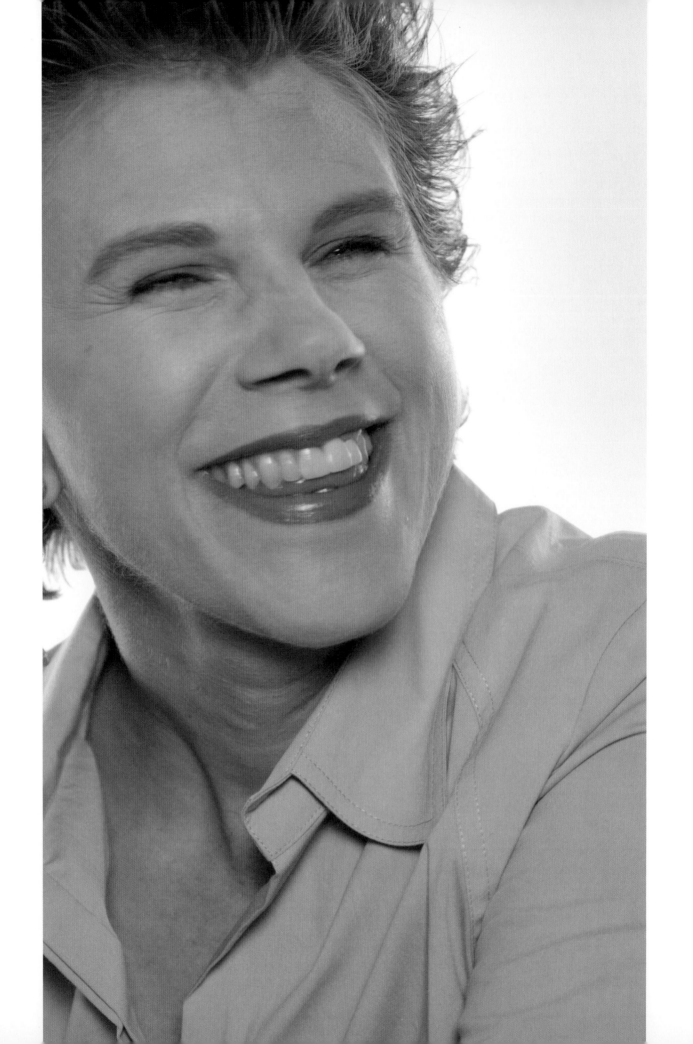

BLUSH

So far, you've used the tools and techniques of skin care to clean and freshen your face. Then you corrected any imperfections, applied foundation, and highlighted the areas under your eyes. Next, you put on eyebrows, restoring the natural hairline of your brows. After that, you applied lipstick so that you really began to perk up your color. Now you're going to add blush. This whole process is designed to teach you application *with balance.*

Blush is not designed to give someone a great big round circle of color. The role of blush is to add color to the cheeks in a way that looks natural. When makeup is done in the order mapped out, with the hue of your lipstick and the tone of your blush in place, you'll see a refreshed, natural look emerging.

During treatment you may notice that your skin has become very pale, sallow, or tinged with a yellow tone. With blush as your tool, you'll be able to create a heightened, natural look that puts color back in your complexion. Success with blush depends upon application and color. You need to choose a flattering shade of color and then apply it to the correct area of your face.

When putting color back in your face, don't focus on blush alone. Instead, think about all the work we've done so far throughout our makeup session:

- Performing good overall skin care techniques.

- Making your face be your canvas, using camouflage, foundation, and highlighter under the eyes.

- Adding powder to keep makeup fresh.

- Applying corrective techniques for the eyebrows.

- Applying lipstick – changing hues; making lipstick last.

- Now, adding blush.

As you can see, we are building up to a very natural, soft look. You can already see the color coming back into your face.

Remember – you *will* get your natural coloring back after treatment. In the meantime, one of the biggest mistakes that people make with blush is to put on too much, trying to overcompensate for the lack of color. You think you need to dive in with a strong blush and end up sticking bright colors all over your face. Wrong! It looks unnatural and artificial.

Instead, use color sparingly and with proper application. The look you end up with will be natural and complementary.

As with all makeup products, there are different types of blush on the market. First, examine what you already have. Cream or powder? What do you prefer to work with?

Powder: My personal favorite. You have much more control with a powder blush. But don't use the tiny brush that comes in compacts. A large brush works much better.

Cream and gels: Much harder to control color. These work best on dry skin.

Combination: If you really have a problem with color melting down into your skin, it can help to use a powder blush with a cream blush underneath. This will help lock the color in.

Other options: Some people even use lipstick as a cream because they like the color. If you don't have blush at home, lipstick can work just fine. Again, the idea is not to rush out and spend money, but to use what you have. Technique can go a long way in making all kinds of different tools work.

"After my close friend Susan was diagnosed with breast cancer, I could not sit on the sideline and watch her and her family go through this trauma alone. All I wanted to do was to be there for each of them, twenty-four hours a day, to ease their pain and to make a difference.

As Susan's hair, eyelashes, and eyebrows disappeared, I watched her go through emotional despair. I wanted to do something to help her feel and look better. I was honored and thrilled to be able to send Lori Ovitz to Susan's home. Watching Lori's magical touch as she brought my girlfriend's face back to life was something I shall never forget!

Women always want to introduce their close friends to one another, but no one would have thought that breast cancer would be the catalyst in bringing two lives together in such a meaningful way.

Through the hardship of breast cancer, three women's lives have been inextricably interwoven. We all are truly blessed: Susan, Lori, and I, individually and collectively."

– Michele Fisher

Blush and Bronzer

Color

This should be a natural tone that works well with your skin tone and the colors of your clothes. It should also complement the color of your lipstick. For example, if you tend to wear pinks, purples, and blues, then pink-toned blush works well for you. If you have a paler skin, you're going to want to softer, lighter colors. A color that's too hot will overpower your skin. If you have a medium-toned skin, colors that are a light to medium tone are best. If your skin is very dark, using a brighter blush is definitely better. Lighter colors would look too chalky.

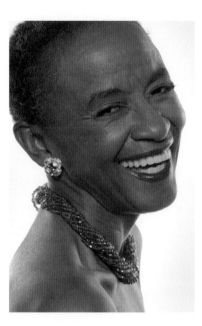

If the blush color you have on hand looks too strong, mix it with powder to soften the look. I like to mix blushes by dipping the brush from one color to the other. You can end up with a fresh new color. Softening colors or mixing them together is a great way to create new colors using the powders you have on hand.

Remember, you don't need to spend a lot of money on blush, so avoid higher-priced products.

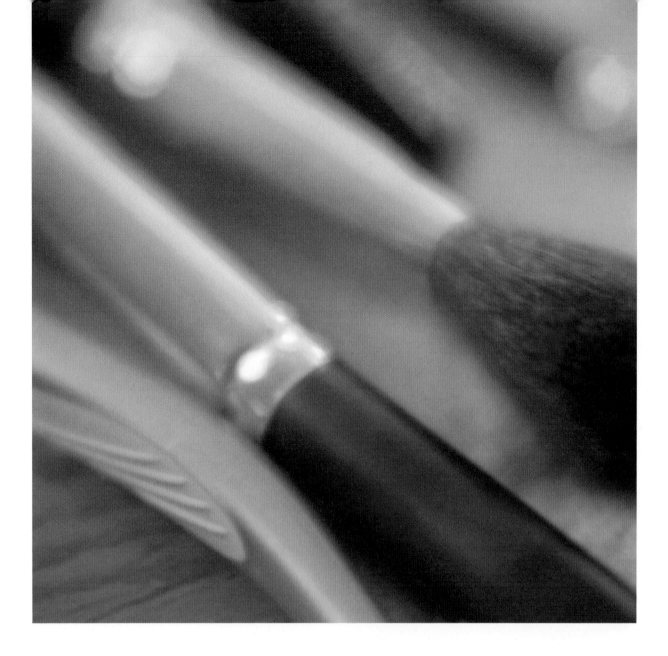

Brushes

Your brush shouldn't be too thick or too thin. Typically, the brushes that come with the blush should be avoided. They're too small and end up making a streaky application. The aim is to have a blush brush that aids in controlling placement and application.

Tip: Don't throw those brushes out, however, because you can use them as a duster to clean up eye shadow or makeup under your eye, or to blend eye makeup.

Where is the proper place to apply blush?

Technique

- Start by looking straight into the mirror.

- Put your fingers into a scissors shape, index finger on top, middle finger on the bottom.

- Turn your hand over so that your palm is facing away from you. Now your middle finger is on the top and your index finger is on the bottom.

- With that top finger, find the top of your cheekbone. With the bottom finger, find the top of your jawbone.

- Between these two points is where your blush will go.

- Recognize the "stop zone": Blush should never be applied any closer to your nose than the middle of the dark part of the eye. And the outside of the blush should never go past your hairline, stopping well before your ears. Particularly if you're wearing a wig, you should not have blush extend into your hair. And a clump of blush in the ear is unattractive.

- By keeping your fingers in a scissors-like opening, with the back of the hand on your cheek, you will find exactly where your blush needs to go.

- Use your brush to swish in that area. Or you can take your hand away and apply blush where you saw the formation outlined by your fingers.

- Never apply blush in a curving motion extending to the forehead.

Remember, if you've applied too much blush, or end up with a color that looks too strong for you, put powder on a powder brush, shake it out, and apply powder over the blush. This trick helps to tone down the intensity of the blush color.

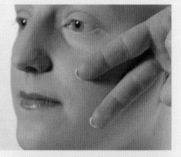

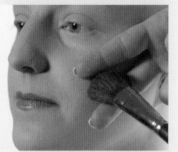

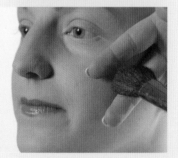

Blush and Bronzer

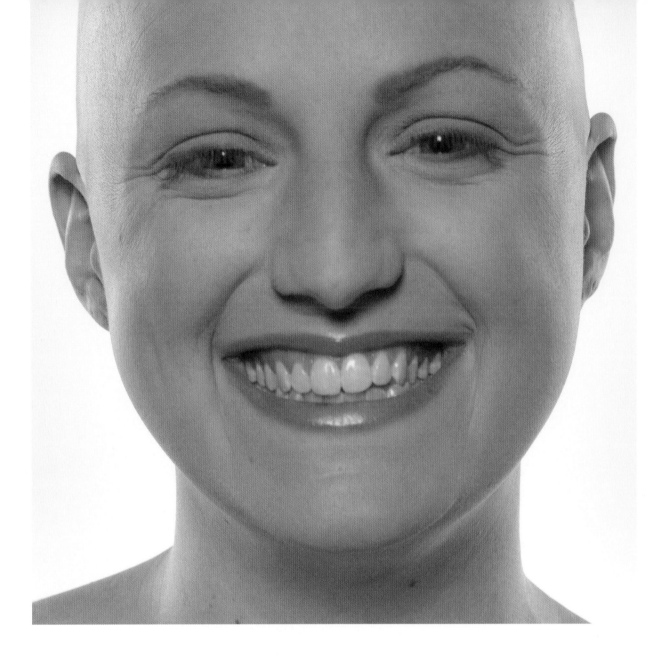

Techniques for Cream Blush or Gel

- Repeat the steps above to find the area between your fingers where your blush will go.

- Place a smidgen of blush on your finger. Make three little dots in the zone between your fingers.

- Using the base of your thumb, press-pat the area you've defined on your face in an oval motion to make the blush smooth.

Caution: Keep the intensity of the color at a level that is natural-looking. Don't overcompensate.

BRONZERS

Bronzing powders and gels are designed to warm up your face with an extra bit of color when you really need it. Also, you can fake a really great tan by using the correct bronzing product! (Just make sure you keep matching the rest of your body's skin tones.) There are many different bronzing products on the market, although some have shimmer in them and others are too fast drying.

I prefer to use a bronzing powder with a big fluffy brush. Bronzers usually come in three different shades: light, medium, and dark. If you have no color from the sun, and if you're fair-skinned, you might want to get a light dusting bronzer and dust it on with a big fluffy brush. Why use a big brush? Because the strokes of a small brush are small, choppy, and blotchy.

Techniques

- Gel bronzers: Mix with a moisturizer to make your application much easier. Apply using long, smooth strokes all over your face. Blend well. Wash your hands immediately to avoid staining your fingers.

- Powder bronzers: Much like applying powder across the forehead and down on the nose, cheeks, and chin. Choose a shade that doesn't have strong orange or red hues, which tend to look artificial.

- Self-tanners: These are not a good option because they clog up the pores, look unnatural, and often have a tone that's too orange. If you're considering a self-tanner, test one part of your skin before you put it all over your face.

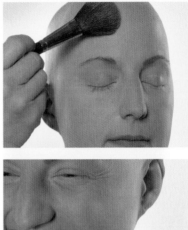
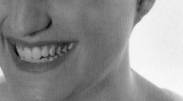

The key with a bronzing product is to make sure it looks natural. Your face should match the rest of you – neck, chest, arms. You want to avoid creating an obvious separation of color between your face and the rest of your body. By applying bronzers properly, you can fake a really good tan!

"My young children never knew what I was going through – I hid it from them. Thanks to your makeup techniques and a proper wig, I could look like myself and not cause them to be frightened about something they couldn't understand."

– Hillary M.

Eye Shadow and Eye Liner

"Finally! A way to learn how to bring my 'self' back."

--Jessica O.

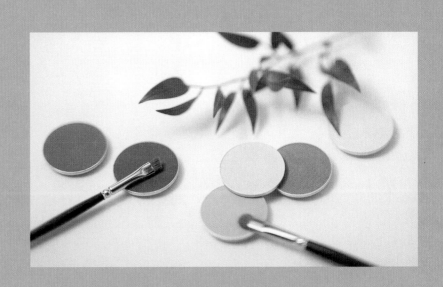

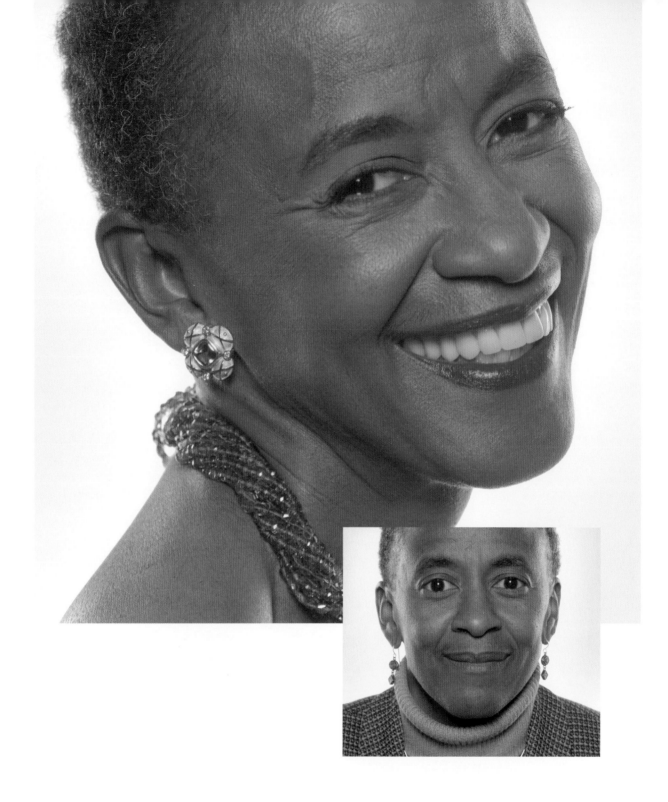

*"Eye makeup works its magic to give the illusion of a
seamless flow of color that brightens and enhances the eyes."*

– Heather U.

122

EYE SHADOW AND EYE LINER

Eye makeup is not just a fashion statement or a trend. Using its tools and techniques, you can correct imperfections and distract from any changes to the eye area. Eye shadow effectively highlights and enhances the color and shape of your eyes. Eye liner has a special purpose – to create the illusion of eyelashes even when they are sparse or missing. The end result is truly flattering. You look completely natural. The colors and lines of the products will not stand out, but the loveliness of your eyes will. It's all about your eyes, not your makeup.

Choosing Corrective Colors

The biggest question is "What color should I use?" The most flattering colors are neutrals ranging from dark browns to creams. You need at least two different shades: a main color and a second, lighter one. By far the most effective eye shadows are powders with a matte finish.

Start by evaluating the colors you already have. Do they include any neutral tones? If you have only an assortment of brighter colors, don't be quick to throw the colors out. Any color can be adapted to a more natural look. If your eye shadow is too dark or intense, change the degree of color by applying a light touch and blend to soften. You can keep adjusting the color until you are satisfied, but always apply each coat lightly, because it's easier to add more color than to take it off.

Neutral tones are best for the basic eye look, but for the evening you can step up your colors by using more dramatic shades. Place a bit more emphasis on the outer corners of your eyes. The main goal here is to enliven your whole face and to accentuate your eyes.

Important Points About Eye Shadow

- Avoid whites. They look chalky and stark.

- Stay away from anything frosted or iridescent. "Sparkly" eye makeup is *not* flattering because the shimmer stands out, crinkles around the eyes, and accentuates any wrinkles. Also, many people are sensitive to its ingredients. Some even may have allergic reactions.

- Dispose of any eye shadow you've had for two years or longer. It's old and can lead to irritation or infection.

Prepping the Eyes With Primer

Unlike foundation or other products that cover the skin, primer is designed especially for the delicate eyelid area. The colors of primer are neutral, and the texture is creamy. Using a primer before you put on shadow serves many functions, such as:

- neutralizing the eyes

- evening-out the skin color

- covering minor discoloration on the eyelids

- grabbing eye shadow color

- giving assurance that your eye makeup will stay put

Once you use a primer for your base, you'll be pleased at how much smoother and easier it is to apply your eye shadow.

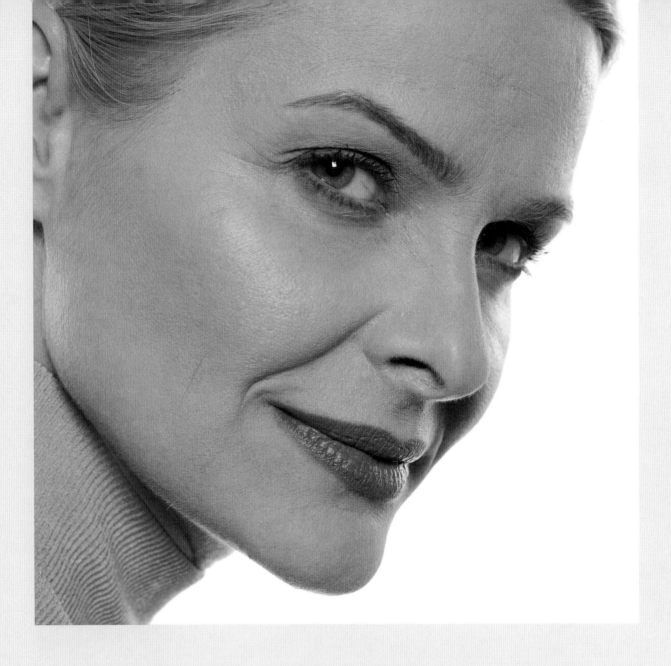

Applying Primer

- Press-pat it with your fingertip.

- Go over the entire eye area, from the lash line to the brow bone.

- Spread smoothly and evenly.

Primer looks so good, you can wear it even without eye shadow!

"I had no idea how to work with the makeup I had at home."

– Tiffany S.

Techniques for Classic Eyes

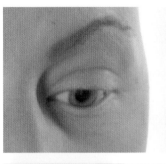

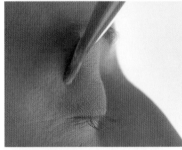

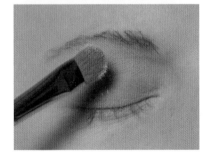

- Using a medium-size fluffy eye shadow brush, apply your main shadow color over the entire eye area, from the lash line to just under the brow bone. Your eyebrows (which you've already mastered) are your guide to knowing where to find the upper boundary.

- Make clean swoops starting from the inner corner of the eye to the edge of the eyelid. Go across in three or four long, flowing strokes.

- From the crease of the eye up to the area just under the brow, apply your second eye shadow. This shade should be lighter than your main shadow.

- Making feather-like strokes with your shadow in an upward direction will naturally blend the products together.

- Blend, blend, blend. You should not be able to see where each of the colors starts and stops.

By following these techniques, you can't miss. The end result looks natural and not "made-up."

Eye Shadow and Eye Liner

Eye Liner

Eye liner is very effective for adding emphasis to your eyes and making them appear larger and bolder. Using eye liner at this time is highly recommended, because it has the unique ability to create the illusion of eyelashes. If your lashes are sparse or temporarily missing, you can learn how to apply eye liner to fill in the gaps so it looks like you have a full set of eyelashes. The end result will look natural.

Note: If you're planning to wear false eyelashes, apply eye liner first.

Choosing Eye Liner Products

- Cake eye liner or eye shadow: the best choices. They look the most natural and stay on well without running down the eyes or melting into the skin.

- Eye pencil: a good choice and handy. But be aware that its lines tend to melt down or smudge.

- Eye liner brush: a small, angled brush – not the one that usually comes with the product. With the right brush in your hand, you can let it do all the work for you.

- Avoid liquid eye liner: This product tends to look unnatural and end up too thick. And it's harder to work with!

Color

The most natural colors for eye liner are dark brown or black. This is especially important if you are using eye liner to create the look of eyelashes.

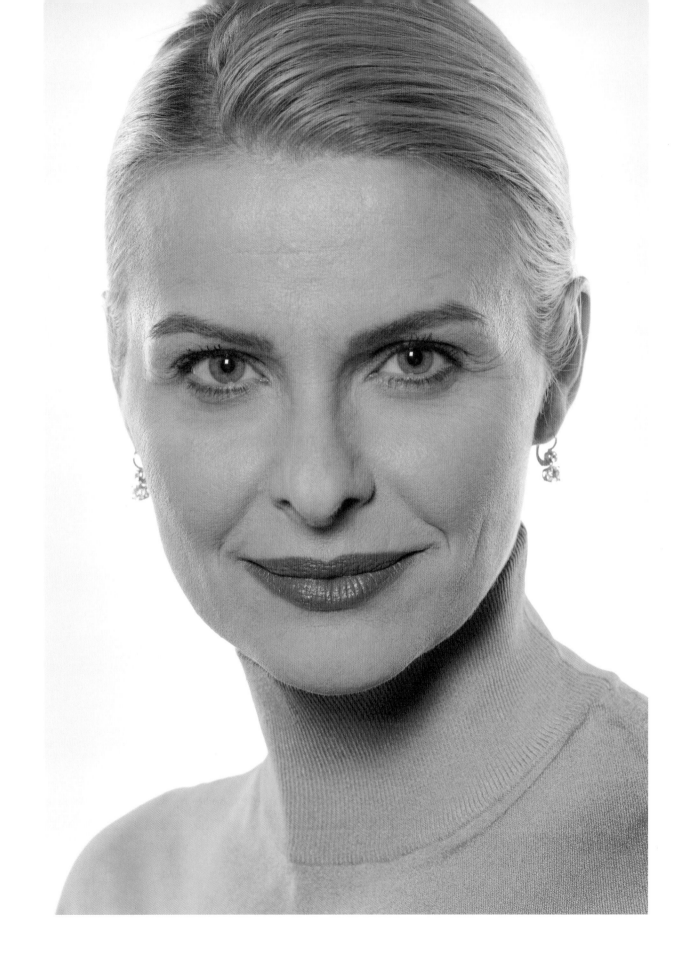

129   Eye Shadow and Eye Liner

Eye Liner Techniques: The Brush Is Key!

- Using eye shadow or cake eye liner: Apply with a damp brush. After you've wet your brush slightly, shake off the excess, and slide the brush gently over the cake or shadow to pick up its color.

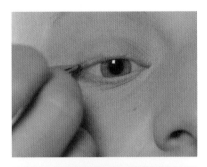

- With a pencil: Don't apply the pencil directly to your eyelids. Instead, use the pencil to smudge the side of your hand. Then dip your brush into the color you've created.

- Bottom lashes: Going underneath the outer edge of the bottom lid, apply your brush right under the lash. Run your brush alongside the line where the hairs originate, as close as you can get. Move the brush gently toward your nose, sliding it half-way across the length of the eye. This light motion creates a very precise, soft line. You can't miss – the brush is doing all the work for you!

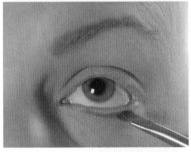

- Using liner to highlight eyes: After you've made the line, smudge the line a little bit with your brush to make it look really soft and well-blended. (Prepare your brush by lightly dampening either the back of the brush or the edge.) This step prevents the beginning and end of the line from standing out too much.

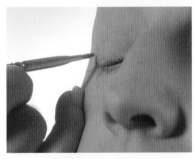

- Repeat application to the other eye.

- Top lashes: Looking into the mirror, slightly tilt your head back and lift your chin up. Look down with your eyes, while still looking in the mirror. At the tilt, you'll be able to see exactly where your eyelashes originate.

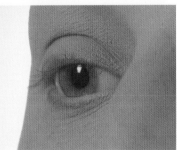

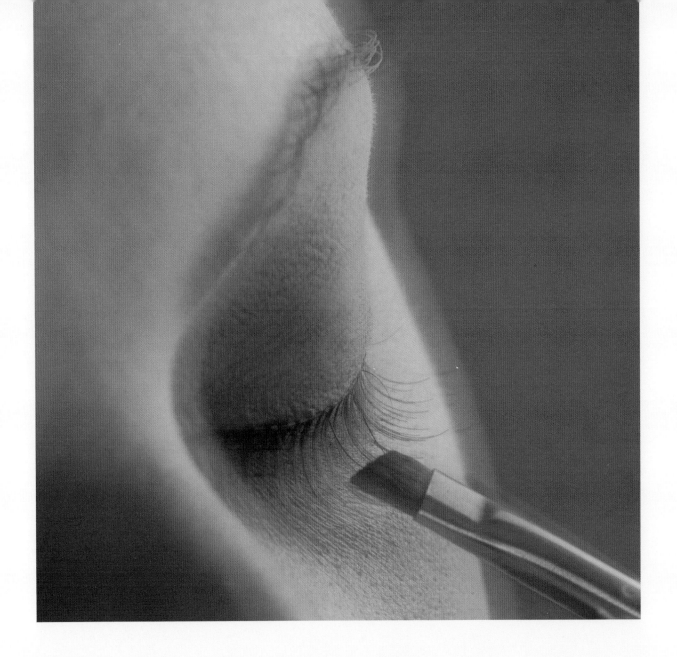

- Determine the starting point of your line – about halfway from your nose to the outer corner of your eye.

- Apply your brush as close to the lash line as you can get. Pointing the smaller angle of the brush toward your nose, slide the brush alongside the eyelash line from the midpoint to the outer corner. Just as on the lower lid, you'll create a precise, natural, thin line thanks to the work of your brush.

- For enhancing the eyes, soften the stop and start points by smudging them.

- For a more dramatic look add a slightly heavier, darker line to the outer corner, and then blend to soften.

Most common mistake: not blending at the end points.

Mascara and
False Eyelashes

Mascara: Color and Application

When to Wear Mascara, and
When Not

False Eyelashes: Techniques for
Full or Partial Hair Loss

*"My lashes and brows seemed to grow back faster thanks
to the illusion makeup provided during the time of regrowth"*

– Kimberly P.

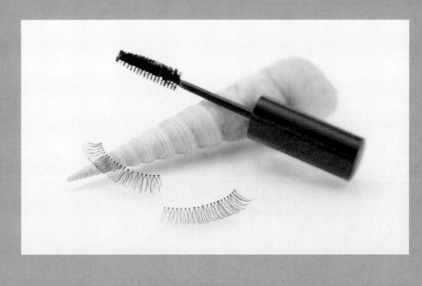

"I never thought I would wear false eyelashes. I was shocked at how natural you can make them look!"

— Katrina H.

MASCARA

Mascara has a role to play in your makeup routine, but it is not recommended when your eyelashes are sparse or missing. Since mascara draws attention to the area, wait until the lashes grow back. When you are satisfied with the length and thickness of your lashes, mascara works well to enhance the lashes and emphasize the eye area.

What You Need to Know About Mascara

- Use only fresh mascara. Start a new tube every two months to prevent buildup of bacteria.

- Avoid daily use of waterproof mascara. Its formula tends to be too drying, and the mascara is harder to remove.

- Treat your eyes gently; they are an especially delicate area. You shouldn't tug or pull on your lashes.

Choosing Products

- Think black. It truly is the most flattering color for all eyes. Browns add too much redness. Colored mascara? Skip it. Any color other than black (blue, violet, red) looks overly dramatic and is a turn-off for most people. (In all my years of doing makeup, I've never carried any color but black in my kit.)

- Lengthening or thickening: Not sure which one to choose? Select a product that does both. Formulas designed just for thickening add too much mascara at once and get clumpy.

- Avoid eyelash curlers: Clamping down on the lashes puts too much stress on the roots. By using your mascara wand properly, you can achieve a look that's every bit as good. If you think you *must* use a curler, be extra gentle.

The most important thing to remember with mascara? Application is key!

Rolling and Lifting Techniques

- Look straight into the mirror.

- Bend your head back slightly so your chin is pointing straight into the mirror. (This is a really helpful position for applying eye makeup.)

- Direct your eyes to look down into the mirror.

- Keep your lids half-open – not totally open or closed.

- Start at the base of the lashes.

- Roll the mascara wand using your thumb.

- For upper lashes, the rolling motion will actually lift and fully extend the wand, letting you curl and coat your lashes.

- For bottom lashes: Use downward strokes on top of the lashes. Apply mascara from the root to the end.

- Apply just two coats. Over-applying causes clumps.

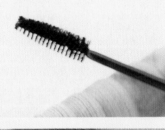

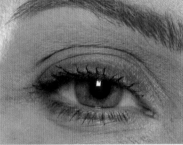

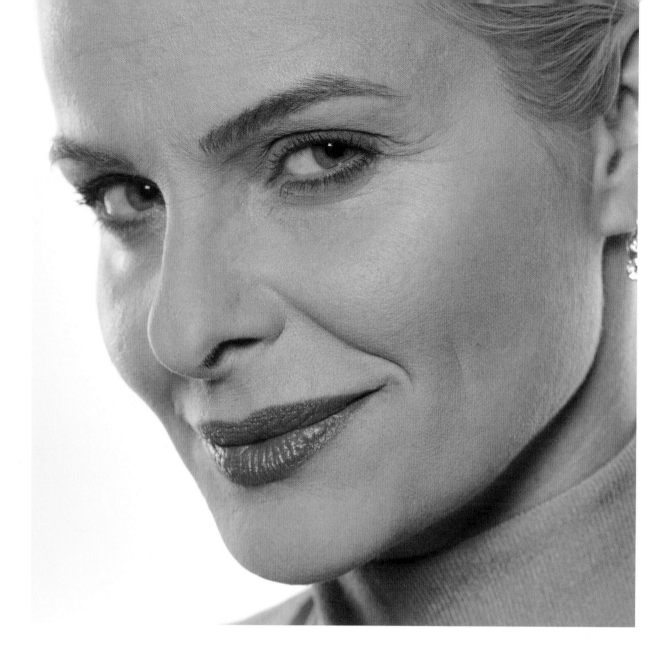

Removing Mascara

Use a water-based eye makeup remover with a small amount of oil in it. A product designed especially for the eyes gets all the makeup off gently and effectively without using detergents or chemicals that are too harsh for the eye. Follow up with a cool washcloth to pat around the eyes and remove any residue. It feels great and is so soothing!

Mascara tips:

- Don't pump your mascara wand in and out of the mascara tube. That motion introduces air into the tube and dries up your mascara.

- Any cleanups (mascara, eye liner) can be done with a cotton swab.

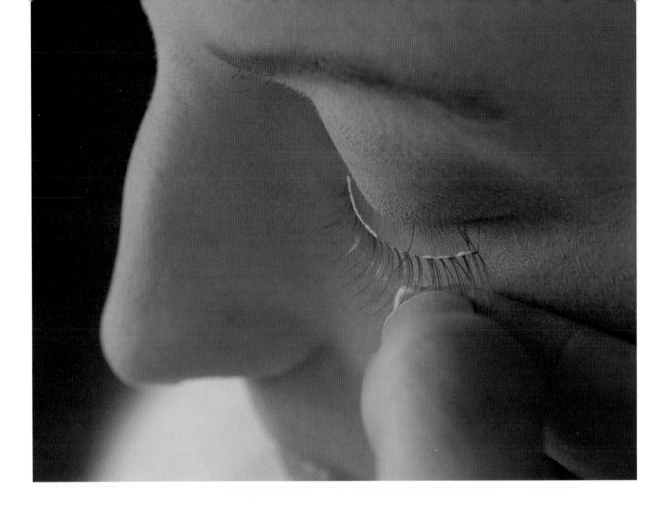

False Eyelashes

Most people don't even consider wearing false eyelashes. If you're one of them, after you learn to how to select and apply false eyelashes you will see that they look totally natural, even if you have no lashes or sparse lashes. You won't even realize you have them on!

There's another big plus to false eyelashes: They're inexpensive, and you can get a really nice looking pair at your drugstore. Of course, if you buy mink-hair lashes, you'll pay much more. But false eyelashes that cost $2.99 can look quite good!

False Eyelashes: Full Band vs. Individual Lashes

Full band lashes cover the whole upper eyelash line. They blend in with existing lashes and cover gaps naturally. Instead of a full band, you can use individual lashes to fill in. These are best when you only have to add a few.

Choosing Natural-Looking Lashes

- Black – the best color choice.

- Invisible bands only!

- Avoid lashes that are too thick – they tend to look fake.

- Lashes look too long? – you can cut most false eyelashes to the appropriate length that's right for you.

Note: False eyelashes are disposable. You should plan on wearing them only two or three times before throwing them out.

Tools for Best Application

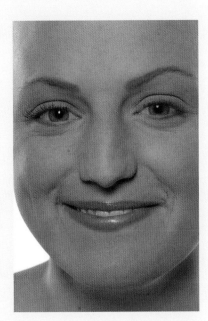

- Small pair of scissors: an essential tool for cutting your eyelashes to size. (Always cut lashes on an angle to customize. If they're too wide, you can snip out individual lashes.)

- Eyelash glue: similar to a surgical glue. Non-irritating, water-resistant, and invisible when it dries.

- Small brush handle or toothpick: for applying the glue across the lash band smoothly.

Applying Full-Band
False Eyelashes

- To keep your hand steady, place your elbow on a surface in front of your mirror.

- Hold the new eyelash between your fingertips, placing it right at the eyelid where you want it to go. Does it need to be cut? Estimate the length that will look most natural.

- Take the eyelash away from your eye. Holding the scissors at an angle, snip off the tips until the length is right. Since eyelashes grow on a curve, don't cut them in a straight line. Just remove a little at a time until you get to the proper length for you. It's simpler than you think.

- Use a small wand to apply a thin line of glue across the band of the lash. Don't use your hand as a palette since glue can be irritating to the skin. Spread the glue evenly.

- Place the lashes slightly above the base of the eyelid where lashes naturally grow.

- Press gently for five seconds. The glue becomes invisible as it dries.

- Repeat on the other eye.

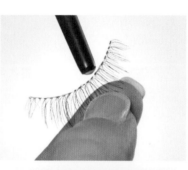

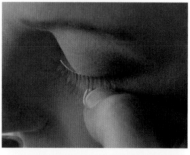

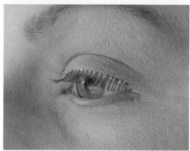

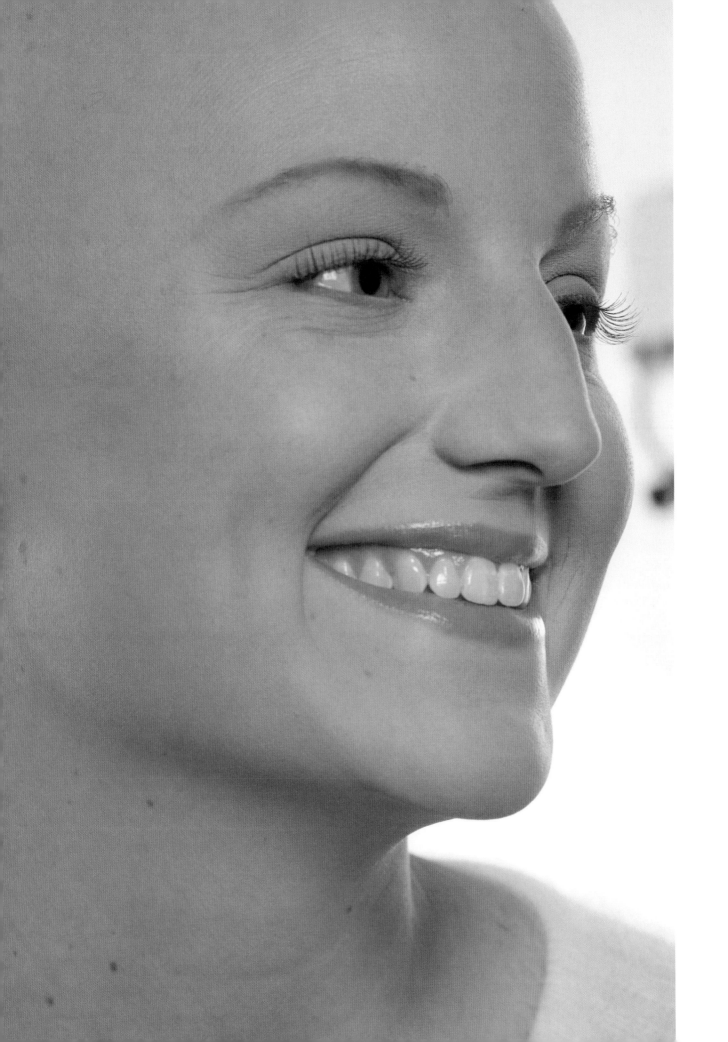

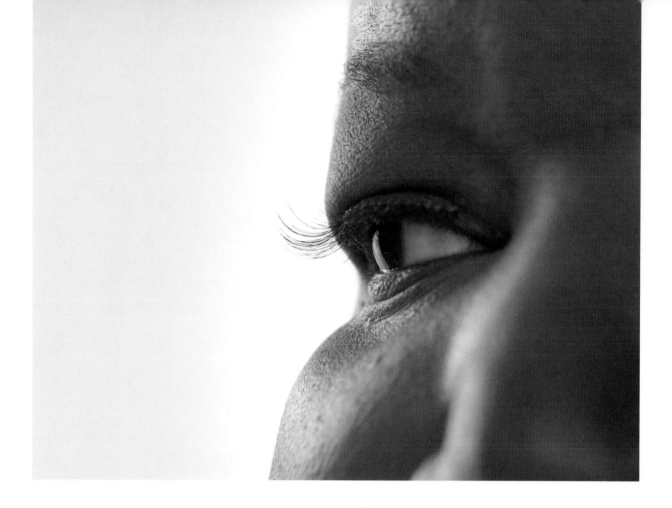

Applying Individual Lashes

- It's the same as applying a full band! The difference is you are focusing on one lash at a time. Measure, trim, and apply glue in the same way.

- Let the lash dry for a few seconds.

- One lash may do the job, or you may need more. If it's just a spot you're treating, use individual lashes. Otherwise, for a broader area, you're better off with a full band.

Tips:

- You can wear false eyelashes throughout the day with total confidence.

- You can apply mascara *gently* over false eyelashes if needed.

- Remember to take your lashes off at the end of the day.

What If the Eyelashes Don't Stick?

- There's too much glue – use less.

- They're in the wrong place – put them in a better spot on your lid.

Removing False Lashes

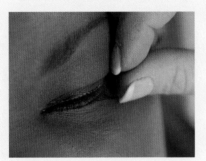

- Gently press-pat your eyes very carefully with eye makeup remover. This will dissolve the glue and help the eyelashes to come off with ease.

- Starting at the outer corner, lightly grab the lashes and gently slide them off.

- Dispose of used lashes after you've worn them two or three times.

"Makeup enabled me to fee

sense of c

over my

— *Jackie H.*

a greater

ontrol

cancer."

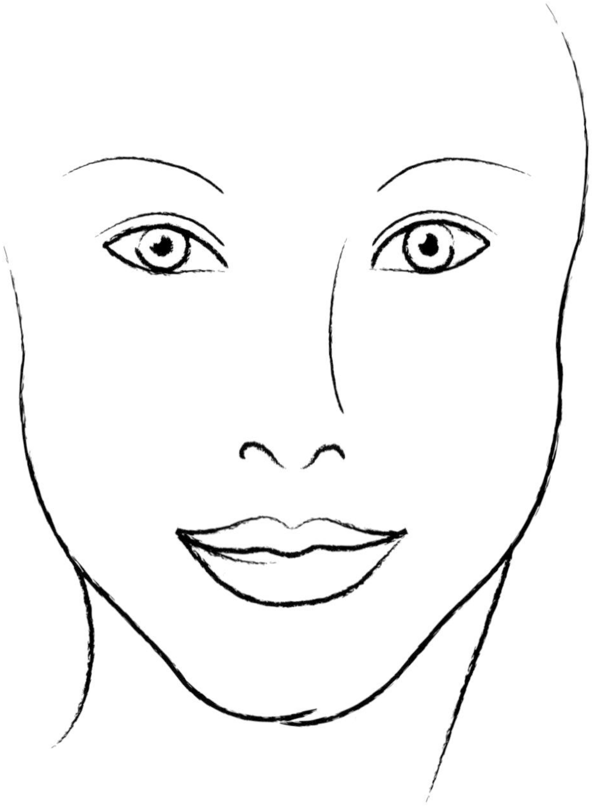

Face and Cheeks

Camouflage

Foundation

Under-Eye Concealer

Powder

Blush

Bronzer

Techniques and Notes

Illustrations by Amanda Onyon

Eyes

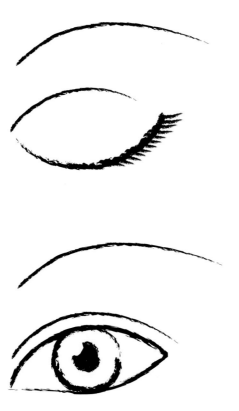

Eye Shadow
_____
_____
_____

Eye Liner
_____
_____
_____

Mascara
_____
_____
_____

False Eyelashes
_____
_____
_____

Techniques and Notes
_____
_____
_____
_____
_____
_____
_____

Brows

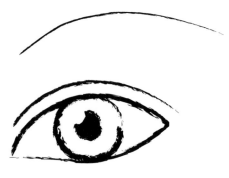

Eyebrow Pencil

_____

_____

Eyebrow Powder

_____

_____

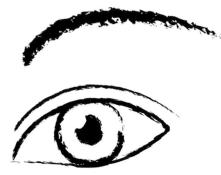

Eyebrow Sealer

_____

_____

Techniques and Notes

_____

_____

_____

_____

_____

_____

_____

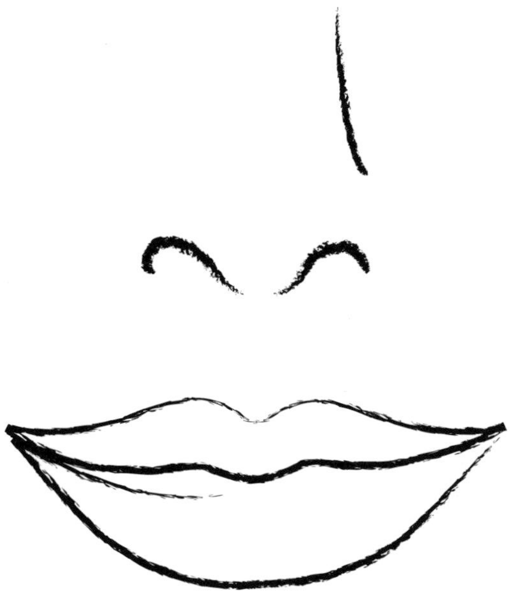

Lips

Lip Liner _____
_____
_____

Lipstick _____
_____
_____

Gloss _____
_____
_____

Techniques and Notes
_____
_____
_____
_____
_____
_____
_____

Part III: From Head to Toe

Wigs

Introduction to Wigs

Questions and Answers

"I've saved a lot of money not having to cut and color my hair – it covers the cost of the wig!"

– Olivia W.

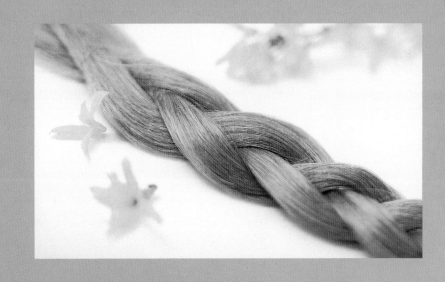

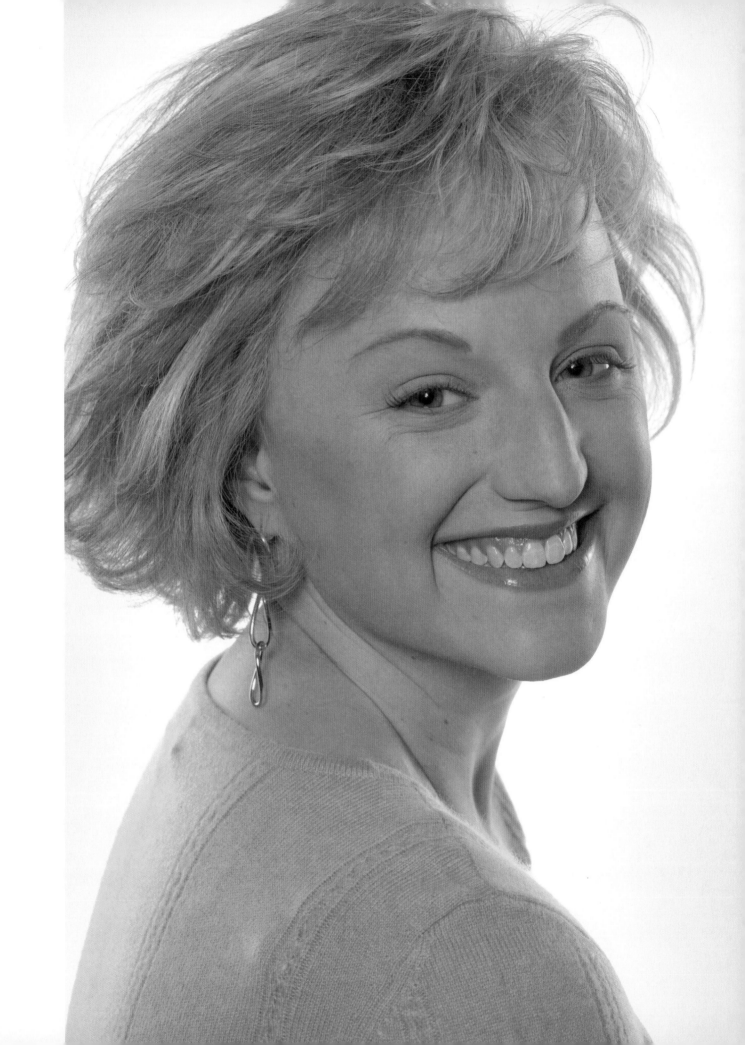

WIGS

Undergoing chemotherapy doesn't necessarily mean you will lose your hair during treatment. Ask your doctor what effects to expect from the type of chemotherapy you'll have. Some people have no hair loss, some have thinning hair, and others lose their hair completely. Coping with the loss of their head and facial hair is one of the biggest challenges many people have to face.

If you expect to experience hair loss, the most valuable advice I can give you is to prepare yourself. Do what you need to do to make the transition easier. Make sure you've made all the arrangements for your wig before your hair starts to fall out. Decide whether you want to match your current color and style, or whether you want to change your hairstyle. Just as with cosmetics, do whatever is most comfortable for you.

Whether or not you've ever thought about wearing a wig before, you are likely to have many questions now. This chapter is designed to answer them. I searched for a top expert on every aspect of wigs, and Brian Blanchard is the name I heard most often. For 25 years, Brian has worked with people nationwide through his Chicago-based salon, Brian Blanchard, Ltd. When I meet one of his clients, even I can't tell if he or she is wearing a wig!

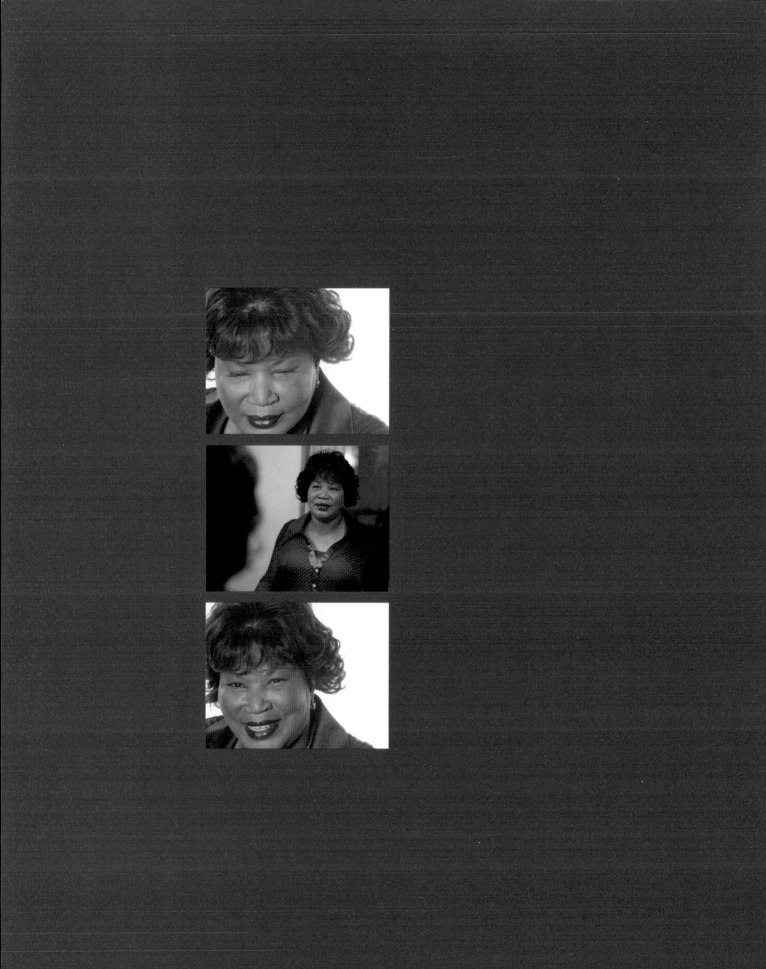

QUESTIONS AND ANSWERS

I hope this Q&A with Brian Blanchard helps make choosing and caring for your wig a pleasant process with great results.

Q: Could you describe some of the characteristics of a good wig?

The best type is a monofilament wig. It gives a more natural appearance because one hair at a time is knotted and applied to a sheer mesh. When you part the hair, you can see scalp through it.

Unless you have a special reason for wanting human hair, I recommend a synthetic replacement. In the past, synthetic fibers felt like shiny doll hair. Now they have been perfected so you can't feel any difference between human and synthetic hair. Synthetic wigs look better and feel better on the head. They are the easiest to care for. About 80 percent of wearers use a synthetic wig. It can be created and colored to match your own coloring.

Another advantage of synthetic hair is that when you steam a curl into it or style it, wet or dry, the curl stays there. After you shampoo it and give it a shake, the style still looks the same. That's what's called "memory." And once it's done, it stays. If you get caught in the rain, you don't have to worry. Water is your best friend with a synthetic wig.

If you're a younger woman who wants hair that's flowing and moves with you, natural hair works great. You can blow it dry, hot roller it – it will act just like hair, and you'll have to take care of it just like hair. Human hair wigs aren't as practical. One example is that they take about 45 minutes to blow dry.

Q: What are the differences between a machine-made wig and one that's made by hand?

Even many less expensive commercial wigs now use monofilament technique for the top. The problem with machine-made versions is that they have "wefts." These are long ribbons of hair that are sewed together on a predesigned base. If you have monofilament only on top, the wefts run around the entire back from ear to ear, and from the top down. They're spaced about half an inch apart, and they have small clumps of hair hanging from the ribbons. When the wind blows or if you inadvertently scratch your head, you can be left with a visible bald spot on the back of your head. These wigs are less expensive because they take much less time to make.

Another difference is that the wefted wigs are heavier, so the machine-made wigs weigh more (sometimes up to three or four ounces) and have more volume. They have so much hair in them! The only wigs you can spot are ones that have too much hair in them.

The handmade hairpieces that we make do not have wefting. Instead, they are hand-tied throughout the entire structure of the wig. You get the same effect no matter where you look at the wig. When hand-tying is done on the full size of the human head, it takes about three weeks for venting, or putting the hairs in – literally one hair at a time through all the areas that are most visible. For the lower back and bottom, they may put in two or three at a time. There are no holes. The mesh is very, very light. Our wigs weigh about an ounce once they are trimmed and styled.

Q: What is the price range for wigs?

A pretty good machine-made wig with monofilament top is in the $500 range. Our synthetic wigs with monofilaments throughout are about $1,200. Human hair wigs are approximately $1,500 depending on the length of the hair.

When you are evaluating prices think about this: If you have your hair colored, cut, and styled on a regular basis, you would spend more than the price of a wig each year! With a wig, you may not have beauty salon expenses.

"A man who sells wigs told me he loved that his wigs allow his clients with cancer to look in the mirror and see themselves first, rather than seeing cancer. Patients have told me that helps them avoid having their whole lives defined by cancer."

– Stephanie Gutz

Q: When should you buy a wig?

Usually as soon as you're diagnosed and your doctors forewarn you about how much hair loss there could be. There's usually a three-week window from the fourteenth to the twenty-first day from the first chemo when hair begins to come out. About 60 percent of people on or about the eighteenth day experience a lot of hair loss.

Q: How do you maintain your wig?

You have to shampoo both types of wigs about once a month, depending on the amount of pollution in the air. You can tell. When the wig looks dull, it is time to wash it.

A major reason why we wash our own hair is because we sleep in it, and it gets messy and oily. Since you take off a wig at night it doesn't get messy in the same way.

You can use your favorite shampoo. I recommend washing a wig with the bathtub faucet because the water pressure is usually higher. The higher the pressure, the easier it is to rinse the soap and cream rinse out of the wig. You may also soak a synthetic wig in tepid water as though you were washing gentle fabrics.

Q: What actually covers your scalp?

Very thin layers of woven meshes are available today. Some stretch in the back to allow for the contours of different heads. The tops are usually a non-stretch see-through material that enables you to see the scalp wherever you wish to part your hair.

Q: Does the scalp get itchy or hot from wearing a wig?

You know the wig is there. An interesting analogy I've heard from a few of my clients is "it's kind of like putting your bra on. The first five minutes you know it's there, and for the rest of the day, it's part of you." It's no different from putting on your shoes and socks or your glasses.

You get very used to it. Wigs today are very light, and they're quite cool in the summer months. In the winter months they play a different role. They become a thermal insulator. As light as they are, they prevent body heat from escaping from the top of your head, and your body doesn't get as cold. Even though your head still breathes, your wig will help to keep your body heat from escaping.

When you first get your wig, I suggest you wear it for a week or so to get used to it and decide whether it needs any adjustments. Typically, I see each client two or three times. The time to make a perfect fit is when your hair is all gone. This is usually done with a slight sewing alteration.

Q: What can you do to care for your scalp?

When your hair falls out you may feel a tingling effect, a slight discomfort that lasts only for a few days. I recommend you treat your smooth head with the products that you use on your face. You don't have to shampoo your scalp. It's just soft skin like your forehead. Whatever is your favorite moisturizer or cleansing cream, just go ahead and apply it to your whole scalp. It keeps your skin nice and soft.

Q: What can you expect when your hair starts to grow back?

Usually, it takes about six weeks for the chemicals to get out of your system and several weeks longer for your hair to begin to grow back. A half an inch a month is the average. The hair usually comes back curly. The pigment and the color are sometimes a little bit different too. It takes about two to three months for the hair to return to its original texture – figure about an inch a month. If you're going to color your hair, I recommend that you wait until you have about an inch of regrowth.

Q: How do you keep the wig on your head?

Make sure your scalp is totally dry. To keep the wig on, use a double-sided, hypoallergenic, surgical adhesive tape, available through wig stores. My preference is a tape made by 3M.

Use a little bit of astringent, like isopropyl alcohol, to rub surface residue off the scalp. No matter how much you wash your head, there will still be oil residue on your skin. Then apply a little piece of tape to the tape tab inside the wig. Usually there are three tabs – one on the top, and one over each temple area. Different designs may have front and back tabs rather than front and temple. Once you've applied the tape, you can work out, ride your bike, do whatever you want, and the tape will hold. You're completely secure even in exercise or high-wind situations. At night, you just peel the wig and tape off.

When your hair starts to reappear and it's at crew-cut length, I switch to small snapping comb clips that are sewn inside, like mini-barettes. They interlock with your own hair. You have to make this change because the tape does not stick to hair, only to scalp.

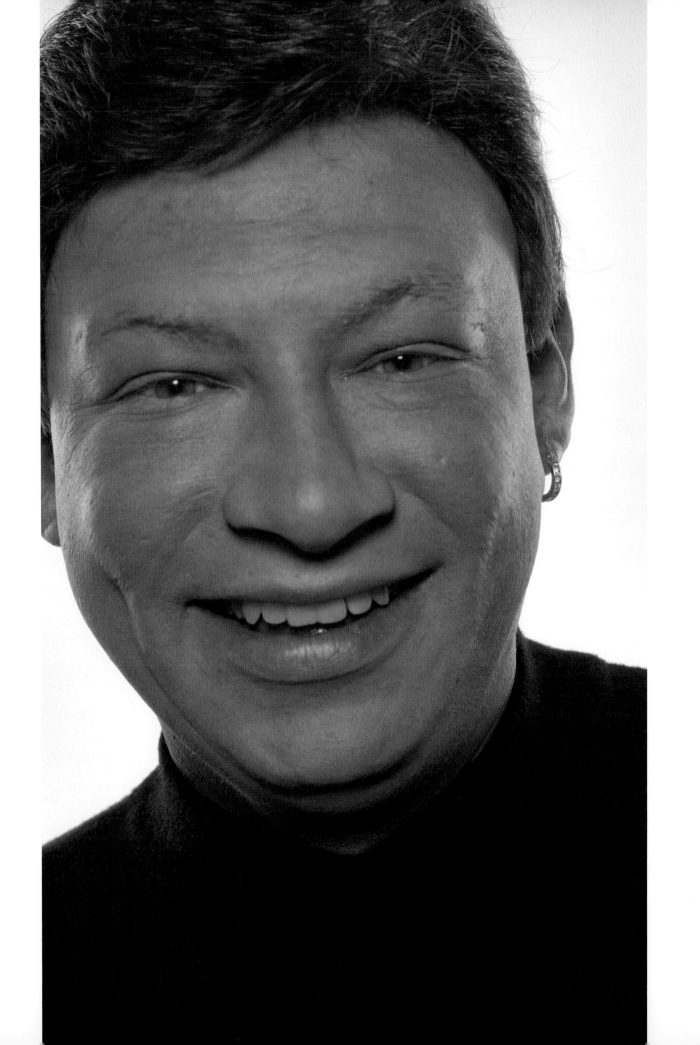

Q: What's a key element for having a hairstyle that looks natural?

When you thin or cut your wig, use texturizing scissors – the jagged-tooth scissors barbers use. They create an irregular soft end when you're cutting the wig and lead to a much more natural look. I recommend using straight scissors only for the final detailing of the wig – to get the right bang length, to trim around the nape of the neck, or to trim any stray hairs that may still be irregular after you texturize the wig. If you use straight scissors in the cutting process, the result looks "wiggier" on any quality wig. Straight scissors make a blunt cut, and the wig won't look as soft and natural. So texturizing is the key to cutting a wig to make it look very natural. If you have any concerns about trimming your wig yourself, it's worthwhile to go to a professional hair stylist with this information.

Q: Are there any cautions about synthetic wigs?

They can melt. They're made of a highly spun fiber that is plastic or a plastic derivative, so be very careful opening the oven door!

Q: How hot does it have to be to create a melting situation?

The extreme heat from the lid of a barbecue grill, a boiling kettle, or opening an oven door can melt the fiber, creating a fuzz. The temperature would have to be over 300 degrees. Make sure you're standing back when you open the oven door to let that first blast of heat out before you reach for your food. After that it's fine. Any normal heat – sun heat, desert heat, normal environmental conditions – can't damage the wig at all. Wigs are virtually indestructible.

Q: Is there anything you can do if the wig becomes frizzy?

If it's just a slight frizzing that comes from excess body heat, it usually can be steamed out. But extreme heat of 300 degrees and above is permanently damaging. That's the only "don't" of a synthetic wig. Stay away from any intense heat. Don't use a curling iron – it's more than 275 or 300 degrees. Professional curling irons can be up to 400 degrees.

Q: What about drying a synthetic wig?

You can use a hair dryer on cool or warm settings only if you have a damp spot. Synthetics dry in about 20 minutes without a hair dryer. The only part of a synthetic wig that remains wet is the nylon or stitching structure on the inside. If you shampoo your synthetic wig and condition it, put it on your head while it is still wet and brush it with your fingers until it looks the way you want it to look, then take it off and hang it on a paper towel roll. It's that easy. It takes several hours for the base to totally dry. The hair itself will probably dry in 20 minutes, but the stitching and nylon on the inside hold the moisture longer. If you wash your wig at night, it's definitely ready to wear by morning.

Q: What is the best way to store a wig?

I recommend hanging any wig on a vase or a roll of paper towels because they don't add pressure that may stretch the inside of the wig when it is damp. If you use a pre-formed wig block made of cork or Styrofoam, the wig can stretch or lose its shape. After several weeks or months, it may not fit as well. People have a tendency to put a wig on a block and tug it down. Inadvertently, they're stretching it.

Another really important factor is that animals like to chew on wigs. In at least six instances in my career, a dog or a cat has chewed a client's wig to shreds. The animal smells your scent, and they're confused. They think your wig is something they should be playing with. If you have a dog or cat, put that roll of paper towels or vase in a closet or in the bathroom and shut the door. Put it someplace where the animal can't get it!

Q: What can you use for sleeping?

To keep your head warm at night, turbans and caps are available in stores and on websites that sell wigs or chemotherapy accessories. Even a paper surgical cap works well.

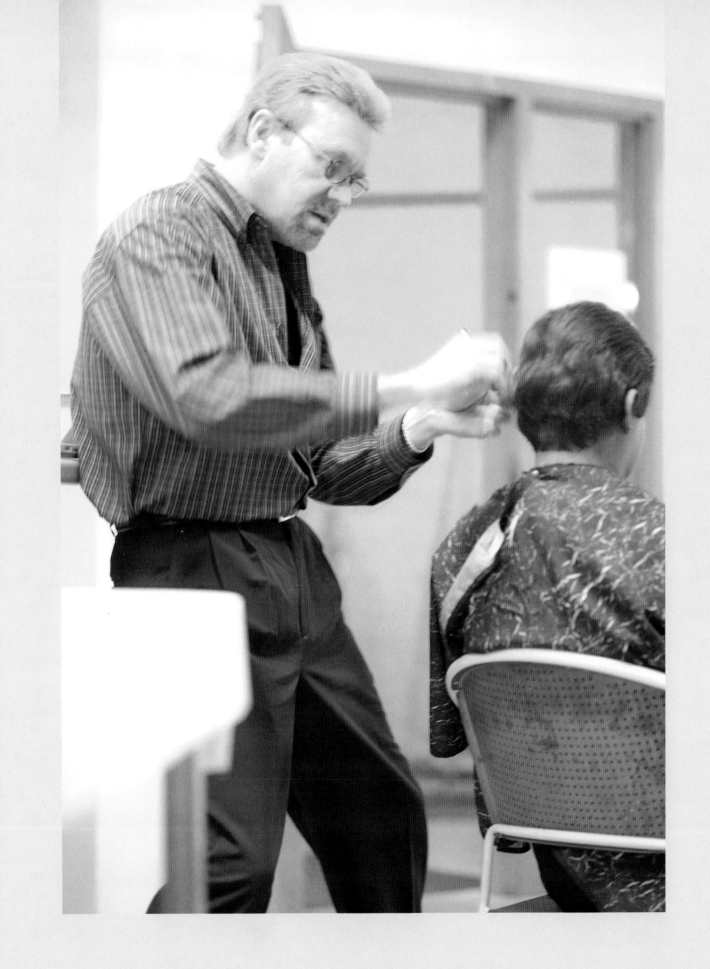

Wigs

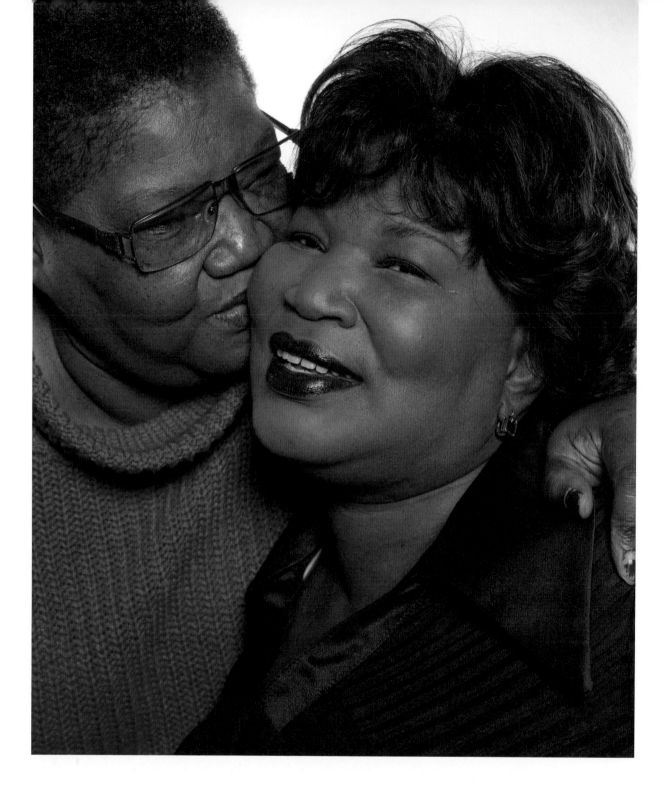

"You made my daughter feel so beautiful both inside and out."

– Lou Emma

Q: What about shaving your head?

Your best choice is to have your head shaved by a professional. Just tell your hairdresser or barber you're going through a temporary medical hair loss and would like to have your head shaved. Barbers and hairdressers can no longer use razor blades due to blood-transmitted diseases, so they have to use disposable razors. A close clipper cut is usually all that is needed.

Q: What about coloring wig hair?

You can't color synthetic hair. It also doesn't fade – a tremendous advantage. Human hair wigs may be softer, and if someone wants a shoulder-length wig they can use a curling iron and hot rollers on, I do sell them. And people love them. But human hair wigs have a tendency to fade over time – after about six to eight months – just from oxidation and UV rays received walking to and from your car.

Alkaline dyes, similar to fabric dyes, are used to dye human hair, and they slow down the fading process quite a bit. But if someone is going to wear a human hair wig for a year or more, it probably will fade a shade or so. Human hair can be low-lighted. We can add a few darker highlights if it gets a little too light. You can darken a human hair wig, but because of the type of the dye and the level at which it easily permeates the hair, it cannot be lightened. When you choose your wig, be sure it is the color you want, or get it a shade lighter so it can be darkened later.

Q: What about swimming in your wig?

I have one word for that: Don't. I just tell people you can look good, or you can swim.

Now if you want to take the kids to the pool and you're in the water with them, and your wig gets splashed and a little bit wet, that's just fine.

Q: Does chlorine affect it?

If it happened once or twice, I would say no. But if you get a lot of chlorine on it, human hair has a tendency to turn green.

Q: Any other exercises you shouldn't do?

No. If you remove the surface oil from your scalp and use adhesive tape, there isn't anything you can't do in your normal life style – jog, exercise, whatever you want.

Q: What can you do when you are done with the wig?

You can donate it to the Y Me organization, or one of the other resources that give wigs to people who can't afford to buy them.

Q: Do you need more than one wig?

Usually, you only need one. If you want something lighter on your head, there are caps available with hair just on the bottom.

Q: Is there any difference in preparing a wig for a man?

It's far easier for women to make this changeover than men, because men often keep the same look for 10, 20, 30 or 40 years. The same haircut, the part in the same place, the same barber, the same style. They want to look the same after treatment. So we have to be really careful about matching the style, matching the color, and making the wig look as close to the original style as possible. Women have much more flexibility when it comes to hair and makeup.

Q: How do people find a wig salon?

Mainly through word of mouth and referrals.

As Brian often tells his clients, don't be too concerned about your hair falling out. Think of it this way – your hair is just going "on vacation."

If you can't make it into Chicago, Brian can usually create the perfect wig for you using several photos and a hair sample.

For further advice, contact Brian at Brian Blanchard, Ltd. in Chicago.

*" ...the best gift **I** gave to myself!"*

— Noreen T.

Fingers and Toes

Introduction

Questions and Answers

*"If I don't take the steps to help myself… how can
I expect anyone else to do it?"*

– Silvia U.

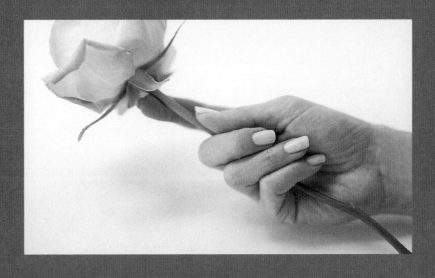

Fingers and Toes

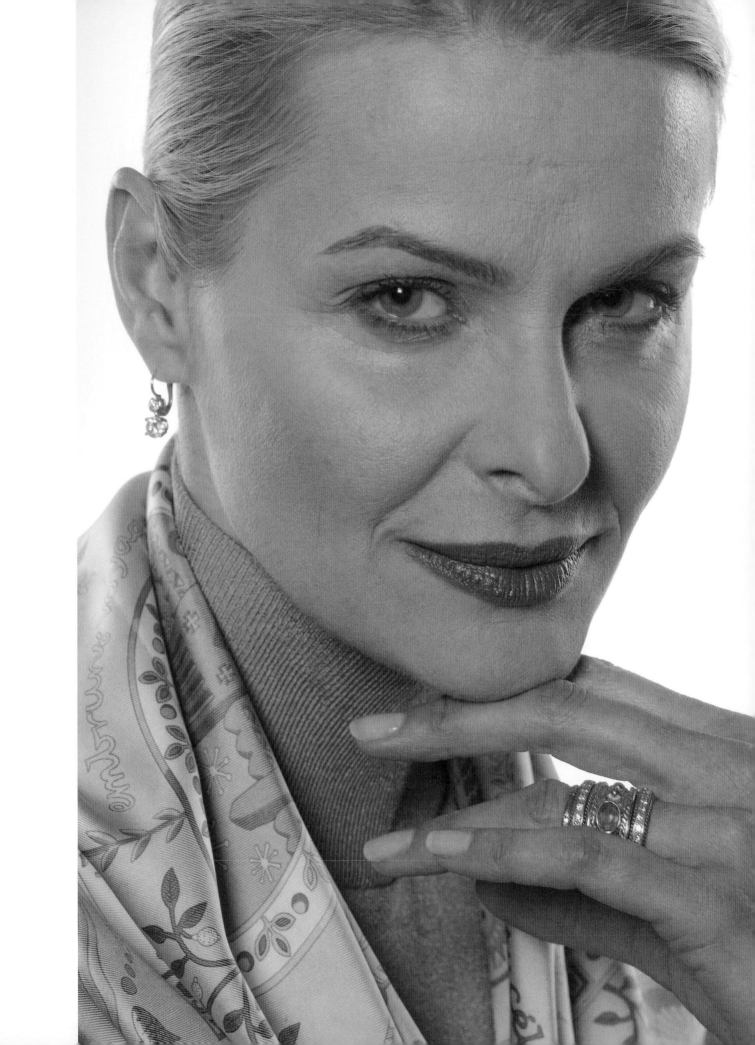

FINGERS AND TOES

Taking care of the skin and nails on your hands and feet is really relaxing and gives you the instant gratification of polished nails and smooth skin. Some people love being pampered at a nail salon by a professional; others enjoy the pleasure of doing their nails themselves. Whichever you prefer – a lot of women do both – there are some basic nail care issues you need to know. Particularly if your nails are undergoing temporary changes from chemotherapy or other treatments, you'll need to know what to avoid and what makes the nails and nail beds as healthy, strong, and attractive as possible.

For insight into these issues, I asked for advice from an expert, Maureen Donlan of All Star Nails in Chicago. Maureen is a nail technician with a large clientele that includes many individuals who are undergoing treatment for cancer. She is very aware of the challenges this can present for your nails and nail beds, and how to take special care with the products and methods you choose.

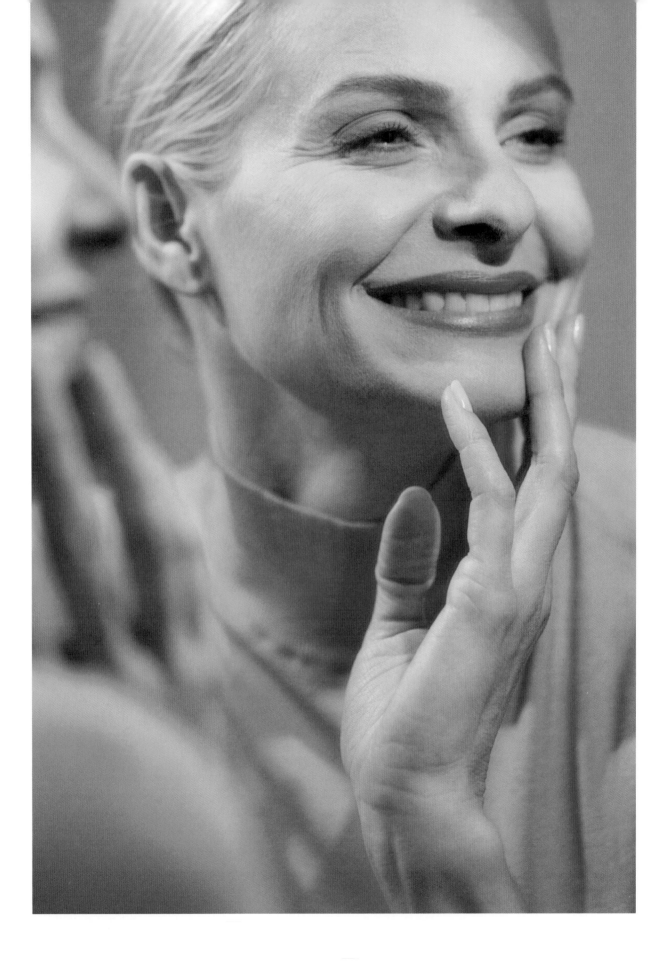

Q & A: MAUREEN'S TECHNIQUES FOR SMOOTH SKIN AND HEALTHY NAILS

Q: What are some important pointers?

- Nail polish remover: Choose only products that do not contain acotane.

- To clean nails: Use alcohol in a spray bottle (there's even a cherry-scented version.) This prevents the polish from bubbling when you apply it and helps it adhere much better to the nails.

- Quick dries: Quick drying helps make the polish stay on.

- Stay with the same brand. It's better to keep the same kind of proteins on your nails.

Q: Besides acotane, what other products should you be cautious about?

One product to watch out for is an acrylic liquid that actually came out of the dental industry. It's too harsh for those who have been through chemotherapy and feel weakness in their fingernails.

Q: Do cancer treatments generally result in nails that are harder and a little more brittle?

I think it depends on what kind of chemotherapy you are having. Sometimes the nails are too soft or they crack. Often, nails have a tendency to get a little thinner. It's best to be more sensitive in everything you do with your nails so you don't puncture the nail or the skin.

Q: What advice do you have for nails that are cracking, chipping, or peeling?

Use moisturizers and buffers to help reduce ridging and peeling. I also suggest clients use a homecare treatment that is very effective:

- Put a little olive oil in a bowl – enough to soak the nails all the way to the cuticle.

- Microwave the oil for about 30 seconds.

- Soak your nails in the oil for about five minutes. This will help give moisture to the nails so they won't get brittle and break as easily.

- Take the pad of your finger and push your cuticles back. Don't wipe the oil off – just rub it into your cuticles.

- After you finish with the oil, use hand lotion all over your hands.

- Repeat these steps about three times a week.

Q: What do you recommend for very dry hands and feet?

Here's my favorite recipe:

- Take a washcloth, dampen it, and put it in a microwave oven for no more than a minute.

- Shake out some of the steam.

- Wrap your hands or feet in the warm towel to open up the pores.

- Remove the towel and apply your favorite oil or lotion. It will really soak in! The moist heat will relieve any aches you might have in your hands or feet.

- Another helpful trick: Moisten hands and feet with a soothing oil like olive oil or a moisturizer before going to sleep. Then sleep with socks on your feet or gloves on your hands. This not only gives added protection but also helps your manicure and pedicure last longer.

Q: What can you do if nails feel weak and thin?

Apply a little gel or acrylic to give strength to the nails (avoid buffing the nails when you do this). The acrylic or gel also maintains the polish so nails can go two to three weeks without having to be redone.

Q: What can you do about yellowing/discolored nail beds?

Use an extra-soft toothbrush with a small amount of bleach to gently buff the affected nails. Apply a protein-based protective coat before applying colored polish.

Q: Is there a difference between a protein-based coat and a ridge filler?

Yes; the ridge filler is formulated to even out the nails.

Q: How can you be sure not to get water or dirt trapped under sculptured nails or nail tips?

The nail technician who applies the tips or sculptured nails should make sure that doesn't happen. If you crack a nail or if the nail has pulled away from the acrylic, these are steps to follow to prevent mold from growing:

- Apply alcohol on the area.

- Use your hair dryer to blow the nail dry.

- Use nail glue to close the crack.

Q: What should you do if fungus has already formed?

If you have mold or fungus, use bleach to kill bacteria.

- Make a mix of 50 percent bleach and 50 percent water.

- Use an eyedropper to put a drop of the solution in between the nail and the nail bed.

Q: Is the bleach mixture too drying for the nail beds?

Always check with your doctor before using a strong agent like bleach. In general, I've found that if you apply just a small amount once a day to kill fungus or bacteria, the bleach does no harm, and it is effective in drying any material that gets between the nail and the nail bed.

Q: How do you care for cuticles to lessen the risk of infection?

Avoid cutting cuticles. Instead, soak them and then push them back.

Q: What do you recommend for foot care and preparing for a pedicure?

- Fill a tub of warm water and add antibacterial soap.

- Soak your feet for about 10 minutes.

- Apply an exfoliating skin softener and a callous remover, leaving them on for a few minutes to soften up the skin.

- When your skin feels soft enough, use a pedicure file to file off dead skin. It should slide right off.

- Dry your feet thoroughly.

Q: Any other points you want to make?

Cleanliness is vital! Sanitizing your tools is a must! Be very cautious in selecting a nail technician. Don't shop by price, but instead by how well a nail technician follows good hygiene practices – otherwise you'll end up paying the price. Be completely confident your nail technician is following sterilization procedures with great care. Even as you're being treated, be aware of what's being done to your nails. For example, if there's a problem under a nail, make sure the technician puts a sterilizing solution on it before touching any other nail. The solution should stay on at least a minute before continuing with the manicure. Basic precautions like these should be followed now more than ever.

For further advice, contact Maureen Donlan, the owner of All Star Nails, at 70 East Oak Street in Chicago.

"Take care of yourself, down to the last detail."

— Loraine M.

Part IV: Men, Children, and Teens
Men

Tools and Techniques

Scars

Skin Care

Hair and Scalp

*"When I walk around downtown, people come up to me
and tell me I look better than ever!"*

— Thomas E.

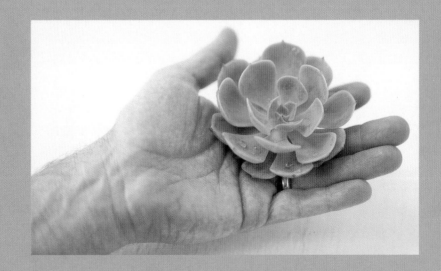

"*When I was diagnosed with cancer, I dealt not only with the emotional trauma of a life-threatening illness but also with some pretty dramatic physical changes as a result of my treatment — like hair loss, scarring, and weight loss.*"

– Lance Armstrong, cancer survivor, champion cyclist and five-time winner of the Tour de France, founder of the Lance Armstrong Foundation

TECHNIQUES FOR MEN

Makeup has a role to play for men. Just as it does for women, makeup can be applied so that it is completely invisible, but restores your natural look as much as possible. You may have to adjust your typical skin care and shaving habits to accommodate the changes in your skin, including increased sensitivity. And if you experience hair loss, there are decisions that you can make on how to respond to that loss.

Skin Care

Dr. Diane S. Berson, assistant professor of dermatology at Weill Medical College of Cornell University, provides ways to treat your skin with special care:

- Shaving techniques: An electric razor is a much better option than using a blade since it reduces the risk of nicks, cuts, and bleeding. If you strongly prefer a razor blade, then be extremely careful.

- Shaving cream: Choose products designed for sensitive skin and rich in emollients.

- Deodorant: Fine to use, but avoid any areas that have exposed raw skin or scars that haven't healed.

- Baths and showers: Keep the temperature mild, pat your skin lightly to dry, and use a moisturizing product on damp skin afterward to prevent excess dryness.

- Sunscreen: Put SPF 30 on the skin whenever you're outdoors. Use a product with both UVB and UVA protection.

For additional skin care tips, please refer to Chapter One.

Men

Harris Jones, 24, cancer survivor and now the sports marketing representative at ALSAC, the fund-raising arm of St. Jude Children's Research Hospital in Memphis, Tenn.

Just a month before I started chemotherapy, I felt as though I were on top of the world. I had entered college after graduating from high school with all the accolades one could imagine, such as being one of only six athletes from the entire country to be a finalist for the Wendy's High School Heisman Trophy. But in that month, my health deteriorated so much I was back home, being tested for what turned out to be a very deadly form of leukemia. Instead of looking at my favorite posters on the walls of my dorm room at Murray State University, I was staring at cartoon characters on the walls of a children's hospital room.

During my eight months of treatment, I learned a lot about myself. Most important, I realized that I might bend, but I'll never break. I realized too what it's like to face the mirror when you are sick. It's the same for guys as for anyone. You think you know what to expect from your reflection, and you don't think twice about it. I remember being in an isolation room – I had been bedridden for some time, and I had to see if I could get up on my own. I happened to catch a glance of myself in the mirror. I didn't recognize my face. In an instant, it hit home for me how bad things had become.

A few months later, my dad and I journeyed outdoors for my first trip outside the hospital in months. A low immune system meant that I had to wear a pink and grey filter mask. These are not my favorite colors. I held tightly to my father's arm as I chose walking instead of using a wheelchair. I began to feel the wind on my skin and realized just how much I missed that feeling. I could see how people – girls – looked at me now. It seemed as if I were a germ, or as if I were contagious. It hurt my feelings so bad. I just wanted to say, "Hey, it's Harris. I was a quarterback, I played college football, I used to be really built. It's still me. Just because I'm 80 pounds lighter and I've got this silly mask on, it's still me!"

Later on, after my treatment was finished and I had been back at college for a year, the doctors cleared me to play again. I wanted it so badly. Facing the mirror then, with my helmet, jersey, and pads back on, was a feeling I'll never forget. I took a look at myself, and then caught a glimpse at all the guys who were standing nearby with their helmets off to salute me as they applauded me.

I come away from my experience at St. Jude with the greatest love and respect for its doctors and staff. They saved my life. And now as I work to help the hospital, I am helping raise money to pay for cancer research and my doctors' salaries, and most important, to help to give children a second chance to live. I have the best job in the world and am honored to know that my efforts in some way help other people. Now, as I walk through the hospital, I see so many kids as sick as I was. And I just want to tell them how courageous, beautiful, and special they are.

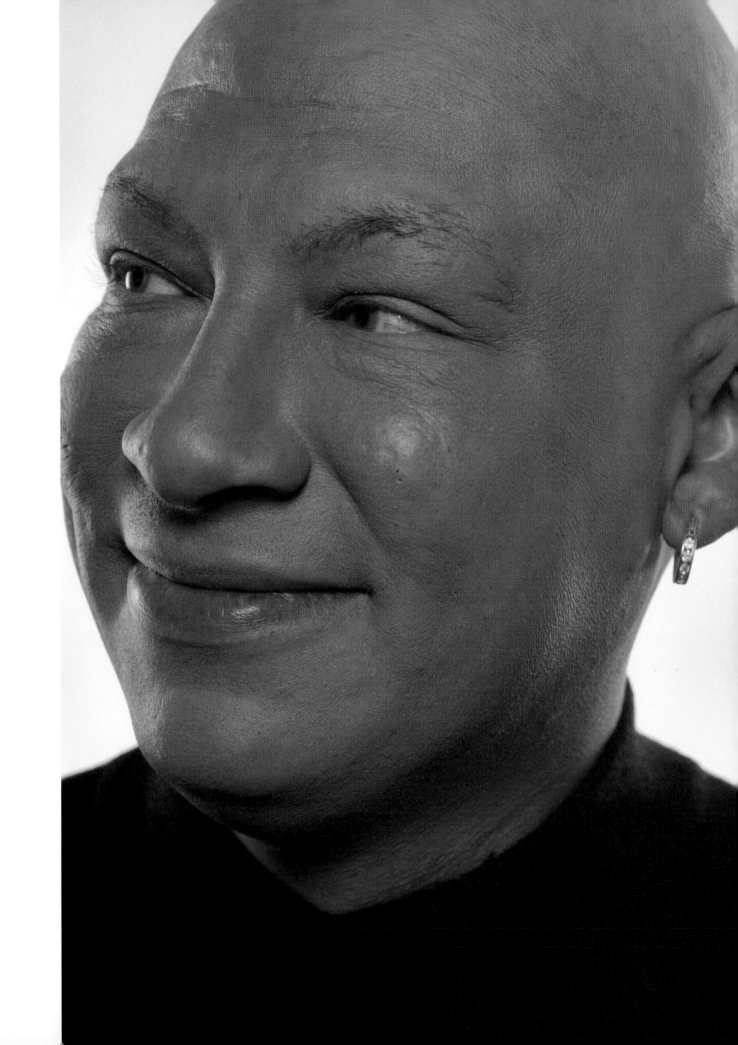

Angel L. Colon, Jr.

First-generation Puerto Rican-American

I want to give many thanks to the Northwestern Memorial Hospital staff and nurses, to Dr. Timothy Kuzel, and especially to Gina Marie Graci, PhD, for listening to me during my many weeks of chemotherapy and for their support and belief in me when I thought all hope was lost. Having gone through what I have, I want to tell all cancer patients that there is a rainbow at the end of all this treatment – the rainbow of life.

Testicular cancer is a difficult cancer, especially because we all believe, "This could never happen to me." I had love and moral support from my family and friends during the good days and bad days, and sometimes there were more bad days than good.

Hair loss was difficult for me. I believed that losing my hair would make people see me differently, but I realized I still looked fine. I ended up liking my appearance – my emotions really were still the same, and I was the same person before and after the chemo. It has all made me a better person, and I now have a different outlook on life.

In return, I would like to again thank all those responsible for my opportunity to say these words today.

Children and Cancer

Dedication

For the Littlest Children

For Kids and Adolescents

For Families

"You made my daughter feel beautiful."

— Heather S.

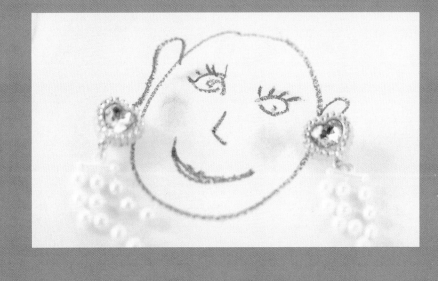

Children and Cancer

"It's an obvious idea, a small gesture, but it's one of the most powerful things you can do. Just treat children with cancer... well, like kids."

– Lori Ovitz

I dedicate this chapter to my friend Sharon: There will always be the most special place in my heart for you. I learned so much from you about courage, strength, and goodness. You have been a very important part of my life!

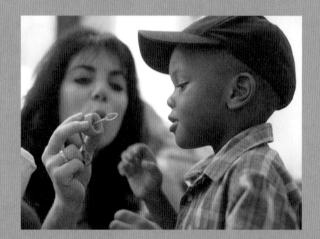

CHILDREN AND CANCER

My friend Sharon was diagnosed with leukemia when we were only 10 years old (and four days apart in age.) I didn't know what that diagnosis meant. I went to my parents and asked them, "What can I do to help Sharon?" Their answer was: "Treat her like you always do."

And I did. We played Barbies, had checker games, ate lunch at the Pickle Barrel. We just hung out. I knew Sharon had lost her hair and that every month she was in the hospital for treatment. As young as I was, I understood the news wasn't good if her mother came back from the clinic silent and drawn.

The one thing Sharon and I didn't do was talk about her illness. She didn't want to, and I didn't ask her. That was nearly 30 years ago, when people didn't talk as openly about sickness and pain as they do today. But what was true then and is still true now is that there was no change in our values. I treated Sharon as the close friend she always was to me. My parents helped her parents in any way they could. Most of all, throughout her four-year battle with leukemia, Sharon's family was totally there for her, giving her all their love and support.

And Sharon was, well, Sharon. Never being anyone but herself. Beautiful, loving, fun, a great student in school, and in religious classes. All in all, she was one tough cookie! She lived her life fully, even when it was throwing the ultimate challenges her way.

Sharon passed away when she was 14. I know her timeless spirit is behind me, encouraging me to bring makeup games to children's bedsides, to write this book to benefit families faced with cancer. I know she would want me to bring this message to the wider world: "Treat children with cancer as the children they are. Play with them to lighten their load. Support their families in every way. Don't deprive anyone one of the little pleasures of life, like a bit of color on their nails, blowing bubbles on a warm spring day, or having a laugh over a silly tattoo."

I think of my friend Sharon every time I go to visit children in their hospital rooms. How much science has advanced in the last 26 years. What incredible strength the children have to endure and to take every possible benefit from the latest research. How wonderful that there are support centers available for educating and supporting parents, siblings, loved ones, friends, and caregivers.

Every child wants to feel special, but no child wants to feel special because he or she is sick, or lacking hair, or in the hospital. My pictures, words, and ideas are here for each of you to share. If these pages help just one person to make a difference in one child's life, then will I feel truly gratified.

*The most giving way to help
children with cancer is to treat them
like you always do.*

Little boys want to show off the names of their favorite heroes on their hats and shirts. And everyone loves to blow bubbles. Or play games. Draw pictures. Wiggle to music. Laugh to a silly story. Those are just a few ideas for bringing love, warmth, and cheer along with you!

Pictures speak louder than words. The photographs on the facing page were taken at a Spring Party given by Facing The Mirror With Cancer.

The Boogie Noogie Spring Fling

Gilda's Club,* Fort Lauderdale, Fla.

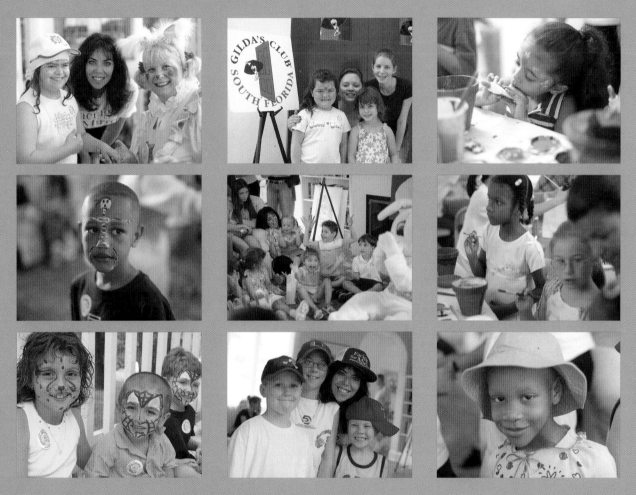

"Living with cancer isn't easy for anyone. When it comes to children and teens, it's the little things that help raise self-esteem and self-confidence, and provide the courage to face the mirror with cancer."

— Trish Lira, Child Life Specialist, Noogieland Manager, Gilda's Club South Florida

• Gilda's Club is a free social and emotional support community for women, men, and children with any type of cancer, and for their families and friends.

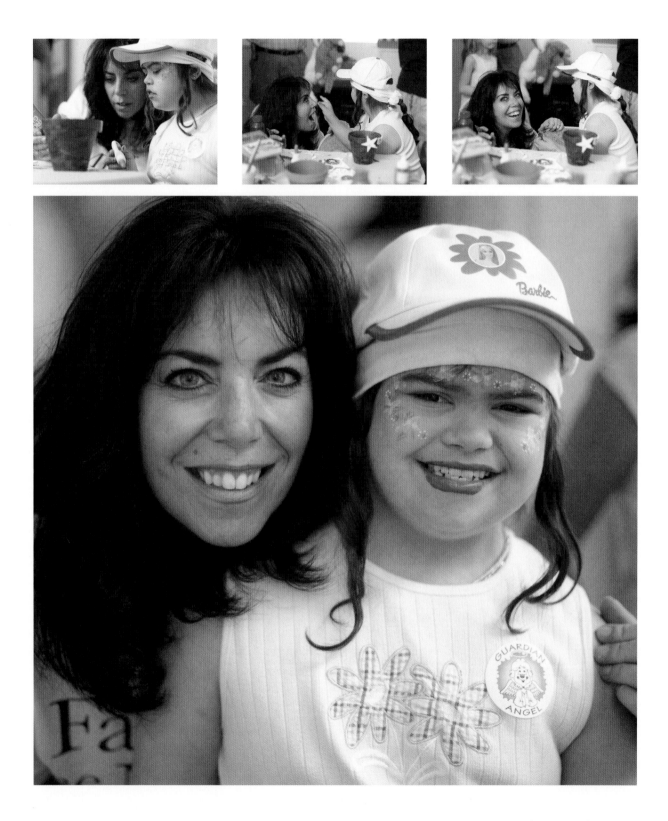

*Parents and caregivers —
don't forget to laugh and enjoy
yourselves too!*

Always treat children's sensitive skin with great care, and be sure to apply broad-spectrum sun protection on a daily basis. That doesn't mean children can't have fun too! Some sunblocks for children are available in different colors. And dermatologist Dr. Diane S. Berson said it's fine to use nontoxic face paint, stick-on tattoos, and stick-on earrings. Have a great time!

Teen Needs

Makeup and Teens

"I remember teaching a 16-year-old girl how to re-create her brows as she was getting treatment. I stepped away from her bedside – and I couldn't believe how real her brows looked! I literally could not tell they were not her natural brows."

– Adrian W.

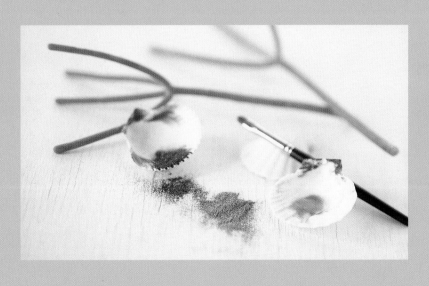

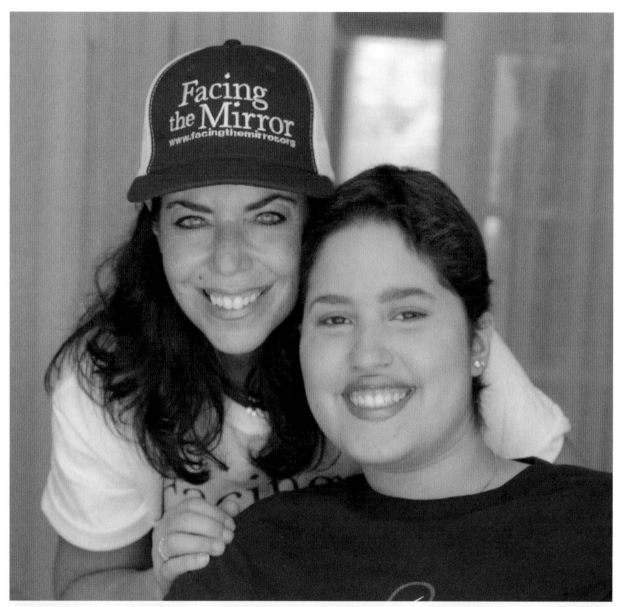

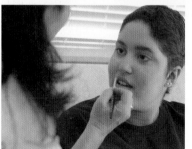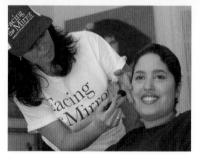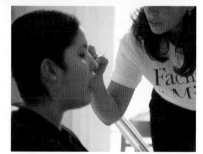

From Chanda Mehta, LCSW oncology,
University of Chicago Hospitals

As a professional social worker, I have had the opportunity to work with many teenagers and children who suffered from cancer. They go through physical and psychological pain that is beyond description. Physical changes include chemotherapy, invasive medical procedures, surgeries, amputations, and transplants, and often palliative or hospice care is needed. The psychological impact of having cancer is even greater than the physical side – having to accept that one has a life-threatening disease. Anger, guilt, bargaining for life, and depression are some of the feelings that are experienced by teenagers and children.

A program like Facing The Mirror, in which Lori Ovitz visits patients, provides makeup tips, and gives individual lessons and little makeup goodies to patients, fills a tremendous need. It gives a simple message of living well with cancer. It helps restore self-esteem and dignity to patients who feel deprived of them.

Teenagers are in a developmental stage in which their bodies are changing rapidly and physical appearance is extremely important to them. Teenagers often feel self-conscious, clumsy, and awkward – and having cancer exaggerates those feelings, since they lose hair and eyebrows, and can start looking older than their years. Whenever Lori has visited our patients for makeup tips or nails, it has always left them with a smile, a look of pride that says that no matter what hardships they have, with a little help they can still feel good about themselves. Developmentally, for teenagers, it has done wonders.

The service Lori offers not only gives them a chance to look better outwardly, but also makes them feel good and proud of who they are. A book on makeup tips for cancer patients is extremely needed since it helps cancer patients learn to accept themselves in a very personal manner. This in turn will benefit the entire family that is battling cancer together.

I appreciate the opportunity to help such a wonderful idea that applauds self-esteem and brings hope to the cancer community.

MAKEUP FOR TEENS

Makeup is fun for all ages, and especially so for teens. You can experiment with color, bring out your features, and try out new looks. The chapters in Part II – "Makeup: This Is How You Do It" answer every question a teen could have about makeup. You can choose the tools and techniques that work for you right now. Here are some examples:

Camouflage: Cover up any imperfection!

Foundation: If you think you need it, here's how to do it.

Under-Eye Concealer: Whisk tired eyes away!

Powder: The light touch to pull it all together.

Eyebrows: Exactly what you need to know to care for full or partial brows, to create eyebrows that look like natural hair, and to smooth out brows as hair grows back.

Lips: Lip gloss, lipstick, lip liner – all the ways to make your lips glow (and how to make great new colors from all the products you have lying around).

Blush and Bronzer: Color – adding just the right amount, in the right tone, in the right place.

Eye Shadow and Eye Liner: Tools and techniques that truly enhance the eyes by emphasizing their own natural beauty.

Mascara and False Eyelashes: You'll never feel intimidated by how to apply either of these if you follow the techniques!

If you are wearing a wig or planning to, be sure to check out Part III – "From Head to Toe." One of the country's top wig experts answers any questions you have.

And what could be nicer than a lovely manicure or pedicure? The "Fingers and Toes" chapter clues you in on the do's and don't's of nail care. Follow the steps, pick out your favorite color, and you're on your way to beautiful nails!

Just a reminder: How you adapt the tools and techniques of makeup to your own needs is up to you. But one thing applies to everyone: Wear sunscreen! For more details on which sunscreen to choose and how to care for your skin while undergoing cancer treatments, please refer to Chapter One.

Check out the beautiful results for yourself!

Coping

"I am more than my cancer, and I strive to live each day to the fullest and accomplish all that I can."

Although living with cancer is an unfamiliar concept, you can look well and live life to the fullest while undergoing treatment and post-treatment. As technological advances are made, people live longer and have a better quality of life. How you cope with your cancer impacts the quality of your life. Being diagnosed with cancer can be a frightening experience and affects all areas of a person's life. However, undergoing cancer treatment does not mean that you have to look like you have cancer or are in treatment. If you can improve your appearance and minimize some of the physical side effects of cancer treatment (e.g., hair loss), you will feel better and cope more effectively with your cancer, as well as with other things in your life.

Always keep in mind that you are more than your cancer. You may have cancer, but you can look as if you do not. An unknown author wrote 10 rules for living with cancer:

It cannot cripple Love,
It cannot shatter Hope,
It cannot corrode Faith,
It cannot eat away Peace,
It cannot destroy Friendship,
It cannot suppress Memories,
It cannot silence Courage,
It cannot invade the Soul,
It cannot steal eternal Life, and
It cannot conquer the Spirit.

Live by these rules and live well.

– Gina Graci, PhD

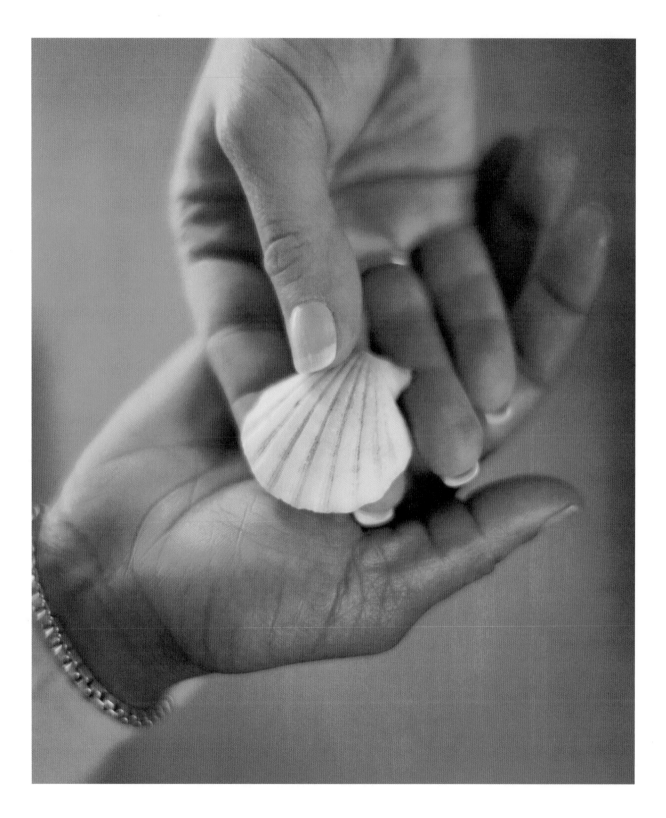

At the end of my lessons I always give
a seashell to my clients – as a symbol of hope
and tranquility.

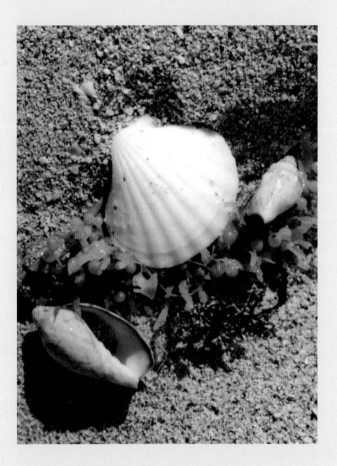

This photograph is dear to me because it was taken by a very
special person in my life.

Photograph by Kimmy Ovitz